Conscious Exercise
and the
Transcendental Sun

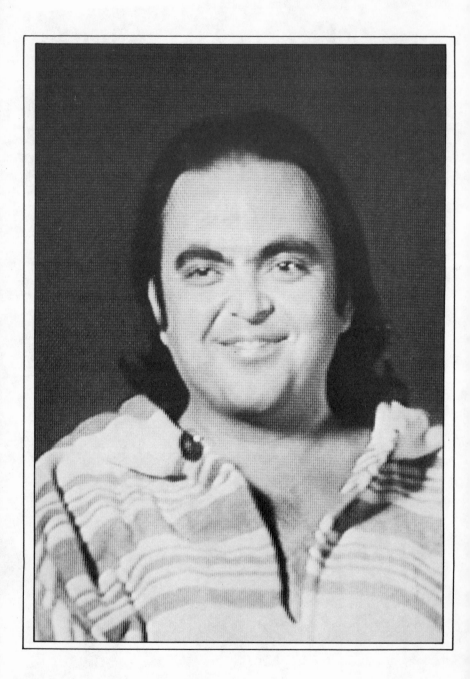

Conscious Exercise and the Transcendental Sun

The principle of love applied to exercise and the method of common physical action. A science of whole body wisdom, or true emotion, intended most especially for those engaged in religious or spiritual life.

prepared in collaboration with
Bubba Free John
and based on his written and verbal instructions

International Standard Book Number:
cloth 0-913922-33-1
paper 0-913922-30-7

Library of Congress Catalog Card Number: 77-83388
Printed in the United States of America

Produced by Vision Mound Ceremony
in cooperation with The Dawn Horse Press

Vision Mound Ceremony

Contents

Chapter 3
The Routines of Formal Exercise   59

Surya Namaskar (Sun Salutation)   80

Calisthenics   100

Hatha Yoga   134

As with any practice related to the health of the body,
it is advisable for all to consult a physician,
particularly one trained in naturopathic medicine,
before beginning any program of exercise.

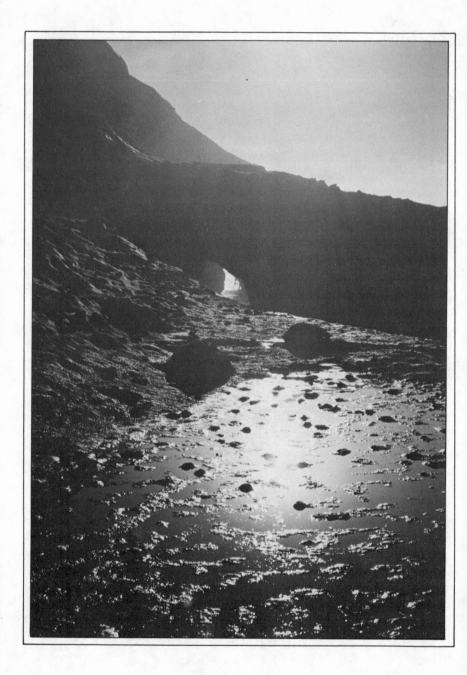

Introduction

The Science of Whole Body Happiness, or True Service: The Unique Approach of Conscious Exercise

Love is the disposition of Radiance, or uncaused happiness in the moment. You always are natively certain of what it would be to look, and feel, and be, and act completely happy in this very moment. Love is to do just that, and to do it effectively toward all relations, whether apparently within or apparently without, so there is no recoil, no separation, no self-definition, but only the Condition which precedes these. Love is thus service, the intention of life toward all natural relations, rather than subjective strategies and seclusion behind reactive attitudes. Love is conscious exercise of the whole body in all relations.

Bubba Free John
The Paradox of Instruction

Introduction

If you can breathe, fully and deeply, and if your breath is consciously attuned, through feeling, to the tangible and infinite energy of the universe—only then can you love.

If your attention is always free of obsession with your own thoughts and reveries and memories and reactions—only then are you capable of genuine participation in life, even in the matters that might otherwise preoccupy you.

If your living body is open, relaxed, fluid with feeling, supple and graceful in its action and expression, and not bound up in a physically visible knot of tension and self-possession—only then can you live a truly effective and moral or relational life in this human realm.

And—only then are you happy.

The system of "conscious exercise" taught by Bubba Free John is far more than a mechanical prescription for breathing or for moving and posing the body. It is a science of total or whole body happiness—a technology of love, or of true service to all beings. The universal admonition to serve or love others is fulfilled through adaptation to the discipline of conscious exercise. It involves a radically new orientation of the individual to unobstructed *feeling as the whole body* (physical, emotional, and mental). It is a foundation discipline not only for formal exercise routines (such as those taught in this book), but for every functional moment of ordinary human existence. One who practices conscious exercise assumes responsibility for his total bodily presence in the human world. And he becomes immediately expressive as a source of energy, life, and light in all relations. Such is true service, or whole body happiness, or love. These terms all indicate what is at once our native Condition and the single appropriate action under all conditions of life.

Most people take up exercise systems (and countless other remedial programs) to achieve, as a result over time, a sense of bodily well-being and happiness. Their motivations are essentially private and self-oriented, even if they hope that their eventual transformation will allow them to become more loving, productive, and energetic in all their relations and activities. But in conscious exercise, whole body happiness is the present and active *principle* of all formal exercise routines and also of every living moment. More than that, as Bubba Free John argues, such happiness, or unobstructed feeling-attention in every instant of relational life, is the principal *obligation* of every mature human being. Happiness never awakens as a result of the strategic efforts of one who is self-possessed. Happiness is identical to sacrifice of self, or love. And love is not properly a goal, but a responsibility, presently and always. The whole approach of conscious exercise is simply an ordinary, pleasurable, and instant way to enliven and integrate body and life-force through the present application of conscious, free attention and intense feeling—and to be expressive to all other things and beings *as* that enlivening force.

Thus, conscious exercise, at base, is a most practical and profound discipline of true morality. Moral action, Bubba Free John shows, is not the suppression or ritual control of pleasure. It is to be so full of pleasure, already, without cause, that you always and gracefully adhere to the universal laws of energy, intimacy, and action. The moral man or woman is not busy obeying societal prescriptions for behavior by suppressing everything in him (or her) that is wild, aggressive, fearful, and explosive with desire. On the other hand, neither does he or she wantonly indulge every arising impulse. The truly moral human being recognizes that we are each wholly responsible for the quality of life that we communicate in every moment, and that we must be expressive in an intelligent and wholly benign way. We must make fear, sorrow, and anger obsolete through the discipline of love in all relations. We must *be* love, if we are to assume full responsibility for our humanity. Conscious exercise makes a science of that responsibility. It fully takes into account the natural laws of body, motion, emotion, energy, breath, and mind, and the dynamic principles whereby all these are focused and integrated from the heart, or the conscious, feeling core of the being. And it aligns all these functions from the heart to the unlimited life-energy of the cosmos: the Transcendental Sun.

As a true Spiritual Master, Bubba Free John continuously lives this whole body happiness or love, in forms of enjoyment and sacrifice. And he simply does not accept the presumption or argument that anyone, under any circumstances, even failure, illness, or death, has the right or proof of unhappiness, or unlove. From his point of view, unqualified Enjoyment, Bliss, or Love is our very Nature and Condition. Thus, the foundation of his spiritual Teaching, which is called the Way of Divine Ignorance, or Radical Understanding, is a prophetic criticism of all human suffering. Bubba teaches that all unhappiness is a childish refusal to participate directly in the whole process of each moment, to love consciously and be already happy and free, even full of energy and life, and to serve or "feed" others with the already selfless radiance of our native enjoyment.

The philosophical and spiritual implications of Bubba's argument are vast and complex. If you are interested in fully considering his spiritual Teaching on Divine Ignorance and its Way, you should consult the principal source books, such as *The Paradox of Instruction* and *Breath and Name*.[1] The present book, which is a guide to the fulfillment of the Law of Life, or Love, in the form of exercise and ordinary bodily action in the midst of all relations, is itself a kind of introduction to Bubba Free John's "argument" or Teaching that the secret of life is Divine or Perfect Ignorance.

The essence of Bubba's argument is simple. No matter what your beliefs, inclinations, goals, perceptions, impulses, experience, knowledge, and activities, in fact and in Truth you do not know what anything *is*—not even your own body and mind, not even your sense of self. For you and every other living being, existence or life is a Mystery, and no one can account for it.

By birth, however, and by all the conventions of human adaptation and education, you are compulsively inclined to react anxiously to this Mystery of being alive. You become and remain self-possessed, inward-turned, a knower, dis-eased in body, emotions, and mind. But Bubba Free John argues that all your ultimate suffering is entirely created by your

---

1. Bubba Free John, *The Paradox of Instruction: An Introduction to the Esoteric Spiritual Teaching of Bubba Free John*, 2d ed., rev. and exp. (San Francisco: The Dawn Horse Press, 1977), and *Breath and Name: The Initiation and Foundation Practices of Free Spiritual Life* (San Francisco: The Dawn Horse Press, 1977).

own presumptions and activities, and, therefore, is entirely unnecessary. You already know what it is to look and feel and be and act completely happy. You can express that happiness at any moment.

This is constantly proven by ordinary men and women. In one instant, an individual may look, and feel, and be, and act unhappy, depressed, in pain, distracted, in-turned and unavailable. But if an incident intervenes—a sudden success, good news, a gift—suddenly he or she is expansive with life and communication. Clearly, that same expression, which looks and feels and is and acts completely happy, could just as well have been generated the moment before. It is simply that we presume to be identified with events, and therefore happiness comes to depend on *reasons* for its expression. But happiness is unreasonable, uncaused, native to us. Fortunate incidents only prove the point. We can look and feel and be and act completely happy at any time. We simply *presume* not to do so.

The true and spiritual Way of life is to be responsible for our presumptions to the point that the logic and script of unhappiness is unnecessary and ineffective, in the present moment, whatever the apparent conditions. It is not a matter of knowing and contracting but of feeling and expanding. It is a matter of being utterly attentive to the whole environment of relations, of things and beings that arise in each moment. It is a matter of the conscious exercise of love, without self-reference. As Bubba writes in *Breath and Name,* it is a discipline of radiant enjoyment:

> Consider what you know. You do not even know what a single thing *is.* Then rest-abide in that Ignorance, as whatever is the case, not *within* what arises, but *as* what arises, as the body itself, whatever is the case altogether

(which is not knowable, but with which one is identical). Rest-abide as whole body attention, not waiting within for changes, but in love. Do, feel this more and more perfectly. Radiate as whole body happiness. Be happy as the body altogether. Look, feel, act, be completely happy as whatever is the case, whatever the body is altogether, under the conditions of whatever is arising. Persist in this under all conditions. In this persistence we are glorified immortally, and the whole future is appropriate, not worthy of fear.

Be the heart. Radiate the whole body. Feel Radiance as the whole body, full of pleasure in the feet and head, the eyes, all organs, the abdomen and sex organs, the chest and shoulders, hands, bowels, anus, spine, forehead, all space, all arising. Be constantly aware of the Real Presence and be submitted into it with every part of every breath.[2]

If you will bring such pleasure and feeling to your practice of even conscious and formal physical exercise, then you will easily become proficient in the way of life-exercise described in the present book. And you will naturally expand healthfully in your practice. Your whole body, including the psychic and energy dimensions as well as the physical dimension, will become more and more radically adapted to the native and Divine Condition of radiant happiness. And you will move more and more naturally *as* love. Conscious exercise releases the chronic knots of self-possession. It unlocks the habitual obstructions to radiant feeling that we build into the whole body through years of reactive living. And it restores all

---

2. *Breath and Name,* II, 7.11, pp. 146-147.

our functions — physical, energic-emotional, and mental — to their lawful conditions and activities as servants of the undefined radiance of feeling that is the heart, or love.

Conscious exercise is an elegant expression of bodily existence. It requires intelligence, emotional sensitivity, and persistent discipline. Every part and function of the being must be consciously re-adapted and re-integrated, through the discipline of right disposition and free attention, to feeling and to the process of exercise or action itself. But the whole process is a natural or lawful adaptation. Over time, without urgency or anxiety, you relax more and more in a graceful, feeling economy of motion, rest, and equalizing rhythms or cycles of breath under all conditions, not only the moments of intentional exercise. The breath deepens, becoming full of feeling, subtle, and exquisitely pleasurable to the whole body. The posture becomes erect and firm, the musculature comes to rest on the skeletal frame, and the whole form becomes supple, strong, and subtly, even visibly, brightened. Undeniably, you begin to enjoy exercise, and every action of life itself, as a continuous link to the Transcendental Sun, the field of manifest light or vibratory, life-giving power that pervades the world and every being. In such a condition you become a sacrifice. You are not busy exulting in any personal transformation or change of state. You realize an altogether different relationship to bodily life and the world, in which you no longer spend time thinking about and demanding attention to yourself, but live unselfconsciously and wisely as a genuine servant of others.

Drawing on Bubba Free John's verbal and written instructions, we have arranged *Conscious Exercise and the Transcendental Sun* in an order that is progressively useful and conducive to practical realization. If you wish to take up this system of exercise, you must first have a clear understanding of its specific principle of action and its basic dynamic functions relative to body, breath, and mind. These matters are considered in chapter one, "The Technology of Love: The Principles and the Process of Conscious Exercise." Then you should begin actual practice by applying ordinary disciplines of right posture, movement, and breath under all conditions, whether standing, walking, or sitting, as described in chapter two. Only then is it useful to learn the brief, formal routines of conscious exercise, including Surya Namaskar (or "Sun Salutation"), Calisthenics, and Hatha Yoga. The details of these routines are given in chapter three. Once you have incorporated all these disciplines into your daily life, you may wish to add a simple, purifying, and regenerative practice of "pranayama," or regulation and control of breath and life-energy, as given in chapter four.

It is not necessary for you to take up the whole Way of Divine Ignorance in order to enjoy and benefit from this sane and pleasurable practice of life and exercise. The essential discipline may be learned by any man or woman who has the capacity to *feel* in relationship, from the heart, with the whole body. The whole approach may be taught, at least in simplified form, to any interested child. Those who follow religious or spiritual teachings other than the Way of Divine Ignorance will find these practices and their specific orientation extremely useful, as they bring to the front the moral energy, free attention, and total psycho-physical sensitivity that are the necessary foundations of any genuine spiritual awakening.

The "science of service" elaborated throughout this book is an especially important consideration for those who are devotees in the Way of Divine Ignorance. For them, the formal physical discipline involved in the practice of conscious exercise is but one of a number of coordinated disciplines that are embraced in life and in spirit. But the core of practice, the intuitive action of love, forms the single necessary gesture that must be maintained and intensified through every stage of the Way. True service, or unobstructed feeling-attention in relationship, is the principle not only of conscious exercise, but of all the practical and spiritual disciplines of the Way of Divine Ignorance. It is the principle of all right practices of diet and health, as communicated in *The Eating Gorilla Comes in Peace,*[3] and of the right and regenerative practice of sexual intimacy, as described in *Love of the Two-Armed Form.*[4] Loving, whole body sacrifice of self is also the principle of all the meditative practices described in *Breath and Name,* as it is in all the stages of spiritual practice of the whole Way of Divine Ignorance. As indicated in both the Epilogue and the Invitation at the end of this book, the focus of devotional practice in this Way is not any manifest experience or change of state or condition for its own sake, but conscious Communion with and, ultimately, Radical Realization of the unqualified Divine Condition of all existence.

Bubba Free John lives as that very Condition. The radiant Sacrifice of the whole body has been his discipline and Realization from birth. His work as Spiritual Master is simply, through criticism, instruc-

---

3. Bubba Free John, *The Eating Gorilla Comes in Peace: The Principle of Love Applied to Diet and the Discipline of True Health. A Natural, Integrated Science of Whole Body Wisdom, Practiced by the World's Great Traditional Cultures and Adapted for Modern Men and Women, Especially Those Engaged in Religious or Spiritual Life* (San Francisco: The Dawn Horse Press, forthcoming).

4. Bubba Free John, *Love of the Two-Armed Form: The Regenerative Function of Sexuality, in Ordinary Life and in Religious or Spiritual Practice* (San Francisco: The Dawn Horse Press, forthcoming).

11

tion, and the transcendental working of his spiritual Presence, to draw others into that same Divine Condition, even during this life. Such is the Dimension of his service to devotees. For Bubba's devotees, all concrete practices, including conscious exercise, are only ways of serving the Spiritual Master and the Divine Reality, in the spiritual disposition of Ignorance, with heart-felt attention, free of obsessive mind and responsible for body and life. All practices are ordinary ways of abiding as a sacrifice to the living fire of Grace. Those who live such an uncommon discipline enjoy the re-adaptation of every dimension of the being, high and low, to the single, unspeakably happy Realization that is God, or the very Reality and Truth of all that arises as experience. The Truth, revealed to intuition, is the Principle and Source-Nature of all existence—even of the Source of light and energy, the Truth of the Transcendental Sun itself.

Middletown, California   Vision Mound Ceremony
June 1, 1977

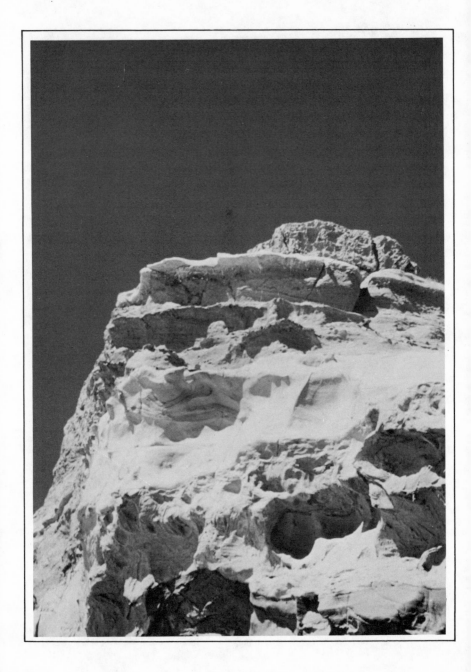

Prologue

The All-Pervading Symbol, by Bubba Free John

The Way of Truth is the Way of Ignorance. In this Way, there is release from subjectivity, from the lie of the inward Absolute, the outer Limit or death, and all the archetypes by which we and the world and the Divine become meanings, like "I" and "Earth" and "God who made us."

Bubba Free John
Breath and Name

Prologue

Consider this. Because we live by experience and knowledge — that is, by reaction — we identify with subjectivity and a subjective or inward self. We think "I" is an irreducible or constant subjectivity — a stream of thought and inner emotion — that causes or initiates actions and speech. Thus, we imagine that "I" thinks, and then says what it thinks. We imagine that "I" feels, and then says or does or otherwise communicates what it feels. We consider ourselves to be an inner being that initiates actions and speech and responds or reacts to actions and speech generated outside the body. The body is thus considered to be the medium between the true subject, or the subjective being, and all that is outside the body. We act as if this were so, and this presumption is the root cause of irresponsibility, illusion, and unhappiness. This presumption is itself the obstruction of feeling, the obstruction of the conductivity of life. It is the failure to love.

If thought ultimately causes or initiates speech, then our notion of a concrete inner self is supported. Indeed, the very reason we are obsessively bound to the stream of subjective events is that we are obsessed with the need to exist and to survive as a specific, concrete *inner* being. The body is made a hedge around the independent inner subject. "I" hides in the body. "I" is hidden from all relations behind the solid, breathing flesh, in a castle tower of thinking and untouchable emotions. And "I" imagines it is the creator of speech and action via concrete thoughts and inward emotions. But is it so? Is "I" protected? Is "I" within?

Notice that at times you speak without thinking at all. There are times — perhaps most of the time — when speech is identical to thought. When you speak without thinking a word before speaking each word, thought does not initiate speech. Then speech is identical to thought. Then thought is speech. Then thought is not inwardness, but action itself.

"I" may become outwardly silent, but thought can and usually does go on. Even so, thought is no different from speech. "I" think and speak. Or "I" *witness* the process of thinking and speaking. Oh yes, and inner feeling too. If "I" write while "I" think, "I" often cease to think first and then write. There is simply writing, which is the same as thinking.

There is no "thinking" that is itself a concrete, independent subject behind action and speech. When "I" am still and inward, "I" may think "I" am identical to the process of thinking. But when "I" act, or speak, or write, the thinking process becomes one with activity — particularly when "I" am most feelingly directed into the process or the relational pattern of action or speaking or writing.

It would seem, then, that when "I" am brought into action most fully, "I" am without any independent subjectivity. The separate, inner initiator of action and speech dissolves into action and speech itself. Then who or what am "I"?

When there is only action or only speech, so there is no separate, inner, thinking me, "I" appears to be profoundly mysterious, shapeless inside, without a place inside, either in the head or any part. "I" witnesses the action, the speech. "I" witnesses the thinking, the subjectivity of concrete emotions and independent states. "I" is even the witness of the thought "I." The thought "I" points to a Ground of witnessing that is not in itself defined, that is prior to the subjective concept "I." The true "I," the Identity of the witness, is utterly unknown, and unknowable, since it witnesses all and is never witnessed. "I" is, prior to its reflection as a concept, the Ground or Consciousness in which the thought "I," and every thought, every sensation, every action, every experience arises. Even the present world arises in such a fashion that it is witnessed by or against this Ground.

"I" think or say "I think," but the thought "I" and every thought ascribed to "I" are all witnessed or intuitively felt to arise within, from, or against the Ground or Consciousness that is not identified or known in itself or concretely over against any thing. "I" itself, the presumed specific inner self, is, therefore, no different from thinking itself, or speech, or any action, or the whole plane of relations. "I" is not inside the body. "I" is coincident with or identical to the whole body, the whole process of the born being and its relations.

"I" is found to be only a thought if we look for it within. But "I" am compelled to think or presume this "I" or separate self. Even so, "I" cannot find any separate self within, any justification for the compulsion, but only the thought "I," and many other thoughts and feelings, which are all temporary and reactive gestures made from past and present experience. Only the "I" thought is constant there. But what initiates the thought? Why does it seem logical?

Clearly, the body is its reason. The life of the body precedes all present thinking. The body is the form that provides the logic of subjectivity, but the life is prior, formless, and unbounded. The life is only made to seem to be identical to the body's limits by association with the cycles of the heartbeat and of breathing. If "I" seek within for "I," "I" find "I" am only a thought, a gesture, not an entity. And that thought, as is the case with all other thoughts, is not caused by any condition that is further within than itself, since only the Ground or Witness stands there where "I" arises and is made a thought. Therefore, the creative source of "I" must be sought in the conditions in which "I" is presumed.

"I" is the whole body talking, referring to *itself*, not to any inward entity. Thoughts are the whole body thinking, not some entity within the body. There is no independent, concrete, subtle, phantom "I" behind and within the body. All that is found within is the spoken or conceptual "I," the whole body referring to itself. Diving within, "I" am led back to my own most superficial form, the whole body itself.

"I" is not the Truth, nor is any of its inner contents. The Truth of "I" is also the Truth of the whole body and the whole pattern of relations—the whole nonsense of all apparent and most obvious and also unseen mechanics, the whole extremity of worlds themselves. The Truth is the unknowable Ground and Field, the very Consciousness, which "I" can never grasp or see but can only be. Neither thought, nor ordinary reactive emotion, nor bodily form is the Sign of it. The infinite life is its Symbol, and only love, or unobstructed feeling, is disposed to the Radical Intuition of the Truth of the whole body-"I".

And that Consciousness is not found exclusively or specifically within or without. Since "I," the whole body, is not identical to its inner or its outer aspect exclusively, but only to itself entirely—the whole psycho-physical diagram or structure or logic, whatever that is altogether—it does not point to the Witness or Condition as either within or without. That

Consciousness Exists coincident with all arising, subjective or objective, simultaneously. It is That of which all arising is the present modification, or on and in which all present arising, within and without, high and low, is a play, or an illusory and unnecessary objectification. That Consciousness, or Happiness, is the always prior and present Condition of "I" and all other arising conditions. "I," the whole body, is That. And since that Bliss is not knowable as some Thing independent of any arising, nor knowable in itself to the exclusion of any arising, it is the Truth, the Condition of all arising, including the whole body-"I". It is Sacrifice or Love. Therefore, "I" is also bound to the same Law. "I" is obliged by the Law of Love bodily.

The whole body is senior to any of its parts, even all inwardness, every thought—even the "I" thought. Thus, prior to inwardness or reactivity, prior to reactive emotions or to speech motivated by thinking, the whole body is alive as attention, unobstructed feeling, and native intuition of its Condition. The matter of conscious exercise and conscious life is ultimately the matter of abiding in the native and free disposition of the whole body, prior to reactions, inwardness, thought, obstruction, dilemma, seeking, and suffering. It is to be present in the infinite pattern of relations with total, free attention, with complete, full, unobstructed feeling, under all conditions. Then there may be the free and sacrificial exercise of life, of love, in all relations, the whole body Radiant with feeling of the Infinite Fullness, and established in Communion with its own Condition to the point of Identity, so there is no differentiation at the Heart of all awareness. Such Communion, prior to all subjectivity or knowledge, and prior to all the effects of "knowledge about," or the experiential familiarity with appearances, high or low, is the Way of Divine Ignorance.

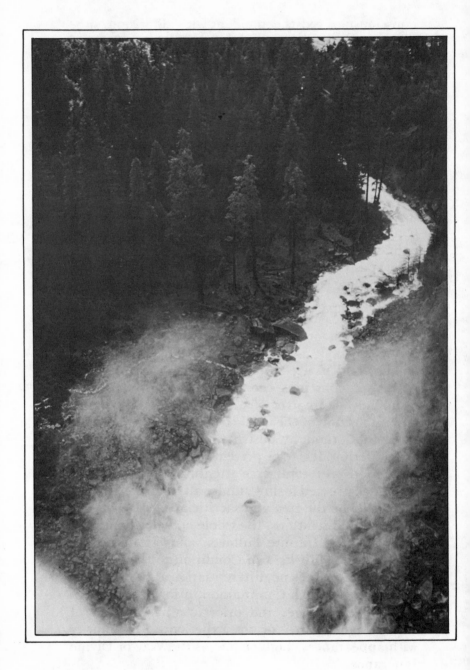

1

The Technology of Love:
The Principles and the Process
of Conscious Exercise

The discipline is constantly, intentionally, and with great feeling to bring the whole body-being into loving, compassionate, pleasurable service and creative cooperation with living beings and whole body (not merely subjective) conditions. It is to bring life-force and body into play via pure attention, rather than to separate life-force and body through a sense of born-contradiction, so that inwardness becomes primary, and obsessive in the form of thought and complicated feeling-conceptions. Love is enthusiastic, humorous, intense, happy, serious, and free.

Love is action. It is not action by an other or a part of a separate one. It is not merely action of body, or feeling, or thought. It is action of the whole body. It is the disposition of Radiance, prior to self apart and all its actions, which are all forms of contraction. It is neither inside nor outside the individual. It is all-pervading. It is the prior Condition of the whole body and all worlds. In Love we are each a living Sacrifice, not a someone trying to survive. When Love is altogether true, when Radiance shines so hard it opens up the hand, then there is only God and God is Love. Love is the Sacrifice of Man.

Bubba Free John
The Paradox of Instruction

1

You may have noticed, especially in most difficult or anxious moments, a persistent contraction or tension of the whole lower trunk of the body, from the heart through the abdomen. This tension often feels like a fist or a stone or a knot, especially in the areas of the navel and the solar plexus. It makes you chronically anxious — not only physically tense, but emotionally, mentally, and psychically uneasy. This tangible disturbance is evidence of a severe and profound reaction to life that is suffered to one degree or another by all human beings.

Thus, the usual man or woman is never happy by mere tendency or conventional adaptation to experience. He (or she) is endlessly lost in thought, scheming, falling into reveries or memories, mulling over the difficulties of daily life. He is at the mercy of random emotional impulses and physical cravings of all kinds. Even his breathing is shallow, forced, and fitful. He is obsessed with power, wealth, relationships, work, food, and sex, the concerns of vital or earthly life. Physical tensions plague him, along with weakness, ill health, and the myriad bodily problems caused by poor posture and self-indulgent habits.

For devotees practicing the Way of Divine Ignorance, conscious exercise and other disciplines serve to prepare the whole being for a profound transformation that makes all such chronic unhappiness unnecessary, ineffective, and, ultimately, obsolete. But for all persons who take up the practice of conscious exercise to any degree, the procedure helps to undermine the grosser habits and reverse the negative effects of the usual life. The discipline reestablishes the physical body, the emotions, and the mind in their lawful, ordinary condition of openness and receptivity to the infinite energy of the cosmos.

From ancient times, the wisdom teachings of esoteric spiritual lore have found it convenient and useful to describe our living being in terms of a series of progressively more subtle bodies or forms: the physical body; the "etheric" or energy body; the astral or lower mental body of gross-level reflection, thinking, memory, and attention; the light body, or the higher mental or intuitive body of subtle knowledge, wisdom, and illumination; and the causal body of primal differentiations, and of the ego, defined self, or soul. In conscious exercise, we coordinate the two lower bodies, the physical and the etheric, through the agency of the lower mind as pure attention and intention. (For consideration of the more subtle and transcendent dimensions of our functional being, see Bubba's principal source text, *The Paradox of Instruction.*)

The Principal Function
of Conscious Exercise

Conscious exercise naturally realigns and integrates the physical body with the etheric or energy body and the universal life-force.

Bubba Free John does not recommend that you attempt, through exercise or any strategic technique, to gain special experience or knowledge of the etheric or energy dimension of existence. If you simply *exercise* in the appropriate spirit and way, you will effectively maintain an ordinary and life-giving relationship between the physical and energy bodie without becoming obsessed or fascinated by either. Simply consider the following discussion of the etheric dimension and body, and then follow Bubba's instructions on the right use of body, breath, feeling, and mind, or free attention, in all conscious activity.

In the physics of the worlds, ether or energy is the senior and most subtle of the gross elements, which also include solid, liquid, fiery, and gaseous substances (the ancient esoteric elements of earth, water, fire, and air). Ether, the most subtle state of gross or material appearance, is the all-pervading element of the physical universe, analogous to space itself. The etheric dimension of force or manifest light pervades and surrounds our universe and every physical body. It is the field of energy, magnetism, and space in which the lower or grosser elements function. Thus, your "etheric body" is the specific concentration of force associated with and surrounding-permeating your physical body. It serves as a conduit for the forces of universal light and energy to the physical body.

In practical terms of daily experience, the etheric aspect of the being is our emotional-sexual, feeling nature. The etheric body functions through and corresponds to the nervous system. Functioning as a medium between the conscious mind and the physical being, it controls the distribution and use of energy and emotion. It is the dimension of vitality or life-force. We feel the etheric dimension of life not only as vital energy and power and magnetic-gravitational forces, but also as the endless play of emotional polarization, positive and negative, to others, objects, the world itself, everything that arises.

We commonly assume that gross food is the principal source of energy for the human body. But in fact the breath is the principal medium of energy to the physical, from the subtle, and gross food is converted at the elemental level through the agency of breathed or assimilated vitality. The breath cycle is the vehicle by which the etheric substance of universal life-force is communicated to and distributed throughout the physical body. When you breathe, you are feeding directly on the cosmic life-energy. Later in this chapter we will indicate how to participate consciously in the process of breathing as reception-release, which is not only a physical but a psycho-physical event of ingestion, conversion, and waste.

Commonly, as soon as people begin to consider human existence in terms of the different bodies, high and low, they become involved in occult and fascinated seeking. They strive to realize their higher or more subtle bodies, to achieve union with them, to attain psychic or mystical experience and knowledge through them. All such efforts are both unnecessary and, ultimately, absurd. They are only motivated by habitual unhappiness, or chronic and reactive contraction of the living being. To the deluded mind of the usual man, who logically presumes that he is limited to what is merely solid and physical, the fascinating and hopeful concepts of energy, mind, light, and "the soul" are fetishes and icons of confused seeking in dilemma. He never sees that his own self-limitation and seeking are themselves only ways of refusing the graceful enjoyment of unlimited energy, light, and consciousness. Bubba Free John writes:

> All life is participation in the condition of Light. Life is conductivity and conversion of transcendent Light. This participation or life is a continuous realization of the condition of relationship or mutual inclusiveness within the vast cosmic process. Through the proper utilization of life-energy and, ultimately, Communion with the Force of the Divine Presence, the devotee is attuned with the inexplicable glory of harmonious existence, which is realized in terms of the functional order or theatre of the cosmos. There is no isolated capsule of force, no separate life. There is only the interplay of cosmic energy in numberless forms of relationship. Through the conscious use of the psycho-physical form and life, or the formal and feeling utilization of life-force, one cooperates in the distribution or unobstructed communication of the infinite force of manifest light, which proceeds from the unmanifest or transcendent, All-Pervading, All-Conscious God-Light. Conscious exercise is a way to enable this cooperation to take place.

Such cooperation is naturally effected when the physical body is properly aligned to and integrated with the etheric. The usual man conceives of his physical, elemental, or gross bodily life as an "isolated capsule of force," separate and independent from all "others" (including the Divine) and the whole cosmic process. He thinks, consequently, that the amount of energy or life available to him is inherently limited. He does not consistently attune himself to the pervasive dimension of energy itself, but confines his attention to the subjective and bodily reflection of it. His anxious and self-possessed way of living seems to validate or prove his mortal point of view. He is only dying. But when we are naturally and happily related to the cosmic energy process through right orientation to the etheric body and its field, we realize that the energy of life is inexhaustible, exceedingly pleasurable, and immediately and always available. The dynamic alignment of the physical and the etheric is, therefore, the effective principle not only of conscious exercise but of all conscious life in this world, including all true healing, purification, regeneration, and positive transformation of the physical body.

The Dynamic Process of Conscious Exercise in Body, Breath, and Mind

These are the foundation principles of the process of conscious exercise:

☐ *free attention,* in which mind is released from random thought or subjective obsession, and made usable as direct awareness and intention, active through feeling;

☐ profound psycho-physical (mental, emotional, and physical) *reception-release* through the cycle of the breath; and

☐ *relaxation-opening or feeling* into the flow and condition of energy as and with the whole physical body, through conscious moving, posing, and repose.

These coordinated principles are, when realized simultaneously, the functional evidence of whole body happiness as it may be demonstrated in mind, emotion and breath, and the physical body. *None* of these functional principles may be true and effective in this sense if the others are not. Therefore, when you exercise in this manner, you are naturally obliged to feel happy as the whole body! And only in that case will you be alive and effective as a singular, integrated process. Conscious exercise is the natural coordination of body (form) and feeling-breath (energy) through free and steady attention (mind).

As you adapt to this way of exercising, you will observe that what you normally consider to be "free attention" is not free at all. On the contrary, the mind is bound to and reflectively obsessed with the experiential sensations and conditions of vital life — past, present, and future. From the beginning of your practice of conscious exercise, you must recognize the tendency to become or remain absorbed in reveries, anxious thinking, and distracted imagining about everyday concerns. When you exercise, either in ordinary activities of standing, sitting, and walking, or in formal routines, allow and intend the mind to feel, control, and follow the body and breath, easily but intensely, as an act of free attention, observation, and responsibility. Do not struggle. You will notice that your interest is always wandering into matters of chronic anxiety and concern. Simply but firmly return attention to the rhythm of the breathing and the bodily moving-posing. Relax the thinking process, which is a form of contracted concentration, and *feel* with the whole body-being. In that case, you will move from a pattern of contraction, which moves toward subjectivity and the specific location of attention in the superficial or thinking brain — and which causes the life center below the heart to contract, or withdraw from relations — and you will instead expand as the whole body into the infinite pattern of energy and relations. As you mature in your practice, your capacity to attend to the exercise process in a simple, unaffected way will become stronger, and the usual, negative games of the mind will cease to distract you so forcefully.

Release all negative, tense, contracted, obstructed, and sluggish conditions of body, emotion, and mind, and receive the enlivening, healing, transforming, fluid, and intensifying force of life itself in all dimensions of your being. This simple process of reception-release is the effective principle in the realignment of the etheric and physical bodies. Even under the best of circumstances, when your own practice of life is perfectly readapted to the Divine Condition or Truth, you will constantly be ingesting or working to eliminate the polluted substances of this world, which include not only physical toxins but psychic and emotional-mental waste and negativity as well. Thus, the practice of consciously releasing all negativity, or the accumulated tendencies toward contraction, and receiving the benign, expansive energy of life, and duplicating its condition in the process, remains a primal responsibility for everyone until this life itself comes to an end.

It is most natural to align the process of reception-release to the cycle of the breath. We already do that, even in our relatively depressed or uncoordinated realization of the life-functions of body, breath, emotion, and mind. Even involuntarily, we allow the force of life to enter and infill the body with the inhalation, and we release at least the physical wastes with exhalation. In the reception-release that Bubba teaches, this purifying process is amplified through conscious attention and deep feeling. With full observation and feeling in every part of the body and mind, feel that you are releasing all thought, all accumulated tensions and negative emotional-sexual conditions, and all toxic substances as you exhale.

Exhale fully, but naturally and easily, with a feeling of elimination from every part and every cell. When you inhale, do so consciously, with whole body feeling, and fully, and allow the universal energy to infill and permeate every function and every cell of your being. Allow the life-energy, which is cycled by this process of reception and release, to permeate and pervade not only the whole body but all arising phenomena, all space. Feel that the force of life spreads through and fills the universe, beyond all that you see and seem to know.

Reception-release, or the cycling of life, is not limited, properly, to the elemental physics of the breath. It is a *psycho*-physical event and action, and it should be engaged at random and often throughout the day, whether or not in alignment with physical inhalation and exhalation. Simply radiate as happiness or fullness of life—physically, emotionally, and mentally. Feel that you are perpetually letting go every kind of obstruction and that you are always opening to and receiving infinite, pervasive, and blissful energy. To look and feel and be and act happy, or full of life-consciousness, *as* the whole body, despite the arising of apparently unhappy tendencies or circumstances of every kind, is itself true and prior reception and simultaneous release.

When body, breath, emotion, and mind are thus naturally, mutually, and rightly engaged, the whole psycho-physical body is naturally opening and yielding to its native and most prior or Divine Condition, not by self-conscious and concerned manipulations, but through generalized conscious *feeling-relaxation*. Even in the more strenuous formal exercises, such as some of the Calisthenics, *always proceed with the sense of the body's deepening relaxation or release into the all-pervading, vibrant field of manifest energy*. It is not by chronic and exclusive tensing of the body that you bring energy into physical life, but by opening it, unclenching it, allowing it to breathe and to move and rest with ease. When we live in contraction, tense, disturbed, motivated to make the body survive at all costs, we resist and minimize the flow of life-force.

To open the body is to feel it as a whole and allow it to rest in its natural state, released and vulnerable in its natural relations, and thus to receive, pervade, and be pervaded by the flow of energy that is always available to it. It is as simple as opening a tightly clenched fist, except it involves not only muscles and ligaments but the whole psycho-physical being as feeling, including the head, the brain, the face, the throat, all bones, the eyes, fingers, feet, internal organs, and also the breath, energies, awareness or attention, even the sense of "me." Such opening is already free of self-reflection, the game of the subjective ego. It is, as Bubba Free John writes, a form of whole body contemplation:

> Contemplation, or bodily yielding of attention into the process of energy, not the physical mechanism in itself or any problem or goal, is the key to conscious exercise or conscious activity in any form. Only then does action or motion of body coincide with both energy and awareness. As the individual exercises, energy is contacted and restored in the relaxed-open state. This process of relaxation and openness of the entire being is to be realized not only in the body, in literal muscle relaxation or no-action — but it is to be engaged in consciousness, with feeling. This is to be done in *every* moment of formal conscious exercise, the purpose of which is to establish *present* adaptation to right, constant, and conscious

involvement with the process of universal energy. It is done by devotion of the whole being to the total exercise process during the entire period of exercise, and during each instant of engagement of right discipline of posture, breath, action, and repose at random times throughout the day. There should be no daydreaming, laziness, etc., but complete devotion of attention through the form of activity. The effect of such exercise is a pleasurable, easeful fullness and sense of well-being under all circumstances of action, as well as the capacity to adapt the being to new and more lawful habits of response and involvement.

The Principles in Action to Which All Exercise and Even Ordinary Activity Must Be Adapted, by Bubba Free John

1. *Do not randomly think and daydream, but apply the mind as free attention to the whole process of the present activity.* Mind is not, in itself, thought. Thought is only one of many objects of attention. Mind is basically consciousness, conscious awareness, or free attention itself. Therefore, the basic condition of mind in any moment is thoughtless free attention, or awareness. If attention is not turned into the relations of the whole body, it will, because of our habitual adaptation to separative and self-possessed games of existence, tend to reflect or randomly turn upon subjective and self-meditative phenomena. Thus, we always think, randomly and obsessively, and we always turn within and away, and we always daydream or meditate on our own sense of indepen-

dent existence, unless we are already and presently turned into the functional pattern of present relations.

2. *Do not merely "perform" actions, as if you were causing them to happen from some detached heaven within or above the body, but feel the entire process of action, with constant attention to every moment of the action.*

Attention is free of thought and all other objects only when it is connected to present events through direct and fully permitted feeling. Attention has no more connection to bodily action or bodily states than it does to the shoes on the lawn, unless that connection is presumed in the present. That presumption is feeling. We may be connected as free attention to whatever objects, functions, or states we may intend, but only if that connection is the one of feeling. Feeling is the medium of relationship. Feeling is the *energy* of attention. Feeling is the life-force. Feeling is our participation in the universal medium in which all objects, including the physical body, arise. Feeling is the whole body intuition of the universal Life and Radiance. Unobstructed feeling is Love.

3. *Consciously, intentionally, as a matter of whole body feeling rather than thought, breathe the constant cycle of inhalation-exhalation as a process of reception and release, and allow it to be timed with the rhythm of all activity, including formal exercise.*

4. *Act, or else be in repose, but always intentionally. However, do not intend only or, in general, at all through thought, or the head alone, but through the spontaneous feeling-intention of the whole body. Such action or repose is always in love, pleasurable, intense, open, and true.*

5. *In summary, always remain active, or associated with the pattern of relations, and do this by presuming the discipline of abiding as constant free attention, through profound whole body feeling*

(rather than reactive or negative and partial-body emotions), in and through the living, breathing, rhythmic play of all functions.

If you will live and exercise in this manner, it will be natural for you to be aware and to feel in and as the universal theatre of life-force, or manifest light. The environment of the *whole* body is not solid, like a wall of concrete pressed against the psyche. When attention is free as present and constant feeling in and through the functions of life, the psycho-physical nature, rather than the merely physical nature, of our total environment begins to become obvious. Then breath and body are realized to be a single process in a single environment, which is made not only of solid elements, but of subtle ranges, including all that may be felt, and thought, conceived, intuited, and realized in Truth. The whole body is the body that includes not only the physical but the etheric, the emotional, the mental, the transcendental, and the consciousness. The environment of the whole body is like the whole body, since the whole body arises from and within it. The environment of the whole body is Light, or Radiance. The Condition of the whole body and its environment is Truth, or the Real. Those who live and exercise in the manner of consciousness, as described here, may also become sensitive and disposed to the whole way of life that characterizes devotees in Truth.

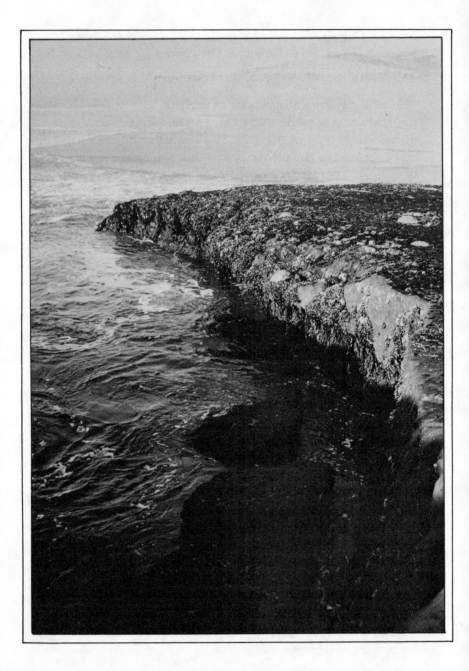

2

All Ordinary Action
Must Become Conscious Exercise:
How to Stand, Sit, Walk, and Breathe

Stay healthy. Do not overeat or overdrink. Do not burden the body with more toxins than it can quickly eliminate. The feeling of bodily aliveness should be constant, under all conditions. The feeling of the strength of life should always be in the navel. Conventional orgasm, negativity, and dilemma (or doubt) discharge the infilled Power of the body-being and weaken it, above and below. Therefore, these must become matters of responsibility as your practice progresses by stages.

Remain in love. Abide as "I love you" under all conditions. Do not dramatize the mood "You don't love me," but remain always as whole body attention, or love, heart-felt.

The head should perpetually feel. The mind is the feeling of Radiant Love, the Bright. Always feel as Radiance-Only, with and as the head, as the whole body.

Throw away everything and be infilled with Living Light, the Perfect and Transforming All-Pervading Power of the Heart, of Ignorance, with every breath. Thus, live by Faith, through natural and spontaneously voluntary adaptation of body, sex-force, feeling, breath, awareness, and attention to the Living Light which is heart-felt to be all-pervading in Ignorance (mental, emotional, sexual, physical).

Bubba Free John
The Paradox of Instruction

2

Conscious exercise is simply conscious, or natural and intentional, coordination of body and life-force, through feeling, in the midst of activity. The disciplines of right posture, movement, and breathing, associated with full and constant feeling-attention, during the natural activities of everyday life are the fundamental regimen or practice of conscious exercise. If you practice intensely, both regularly and at random, you should be able to become proficient in these elementary disciplines within a week or two. Only then should you begin to learn and practice the formal routines of conscious exercise, as taught in chapter three. As the foundation disciplines become more natural to you, you will find that they serve as a continuous form of exercise, a constant reminder and reestablishment of the lawful relationship between the physical body and the life-force, or the elemental and etheric dimensions of the being.

These primary disciplines are the best indication of just how ordinary or common to the whole of life is this practice of conscious exercise. There is nothing fascinating about correcting your posture, about relearning the most mundane forms of action—how to stand, how to sit, how to walk, how to rest, even how to breathe. Especially at the beginning, to perform these practices generates a continual and most unwelcome frustration of the usual bodily habits, and it awakens all the non-glamorous self-knowledge about the laziness and constriction of the whole psychophysical system that such habits perpetuate. This process of re-adaptation may even cause some physical discomfort and pain. Bubba Free John writes:

> The usual activity of most men and women involves a compulsive breaking and obstructing of the life-current, thus creating tensions and inharmonies within the body. Whether acting or at rest, we are usually involved in an endless ritual of twitching and shifting of the body, always compensating for the pain and discomfort of our habitual condition. Through the conscious use of the body, while being randomly mindful of bodily movement and posture, and performing appropriate exercise, one is able to observe and understand the ritual of bodily compensations and pass beyond them into a stable, harmonious condition. Therefore, learn to use the whole body consciously and intuitively in ordinary life and meditation.

How to Stand, Sit, and Walk

There is a fundamental posture appropriate for the human body. Erect, firm and yet flexible, this posture rests the muscles and internal organs on the skeletal frame and maintains all the vital and etheric channels of the respiratory, circulatory, and nervous systems in their natural and most functional conditions. Thus, this fundamental posture allows the entire body-being to receive and conduct the flow of life-energy without obstruction in the midst of all standing, walking, and sitting. It is the structural foundation not only for these ordinary actions, but for all conscious bodily activity, including the poses and movements of formal exercise routines.

When aligned to its native structure, the physical body is supported on the vertical axis by the spine and on the horizontal axis by the pelvis. The pelvis should be perpendicular to the spine and directly underneath the trunk, so that the weight of the upper body is evenly supported by the pelvic bone-structure and both legs.

The pelvis is like a bowl. If you examine the posture of the usual man or woman, you will rarely see anyone in whom the "bowl" is upright or level from front to back. But this upright position of the pelvis, perpendicular to the spine, is the natural position for supporting the weight of the body.

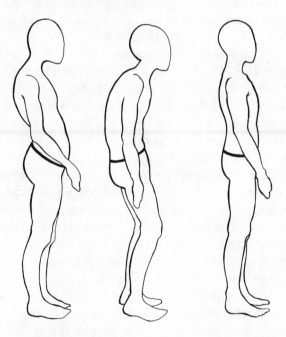

To align the body properly for all standing, walking, and sitting, practice the following simple disciplines:

Standing

A. Stand erect. *Imagine and feel that you are holding a coin between the buttocks without the aid of your hands.* In order to hold the coin you must bring the pelvis forward and up in the front—that is, into a position at a right angle to the spine and directly underneath the upper body. When you move into this position, you will feel the buttocks tuck under the body, and the small of the back will flatten.

B. *Hold the chest high.* When you bring the chest up, the shoulders and upper areas of the body will move naturally into alignment. Do not try to maintain correct posture by holding the shoulders back and up in exaggerated military style. That approach, though commonly suggested, is incorrect; it only fixes the body into a new form of tension and wrong alignment. The shoulders will assume their natural, erect, easeful position when you bring the chest up.

C. *Lightly stretch or extend the spinal column between the "flat" of the lower back (the area where the spine and the pelvis meet) and the top of the head.* Feel as if the body is hanging on the spine, and the spine in turn is hanging from the indentation in the skull to the rear of the middle of the crown. *Learn to relax the neck and the spine under all conditions, while also keeping them lightly but fully extended.* If you direct attention to this relaxing and extending of the spine, the rest of the body will come into natural alignment of its own accord. This relaxing-extending stimulates and enlivens the entire nervous system, bringing it into full, unobstructed contact with the all-pervading life-force. When this alignment is maintained, the head is held erect and rests squarely on the spinal column, which feels as if it were being stretched or pulled from one end to the other. This position may feel uncomfortable or unnatural at first, and you may experience some tension in the lower back, which should always remain nearly flat.

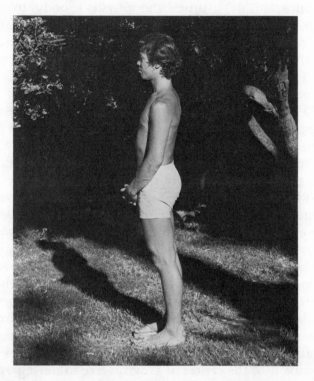

The exaggerated curvature in the lower back, either outward or inward, that is common to most people today causes tension and obstruction of energy to accumulate in that area. Such wrong alignment makes the lower back chronically weak and contributes to many other psycho-physiological difficulties. But the restorative and regenerative effects of assuming and maintaining the appropriate posture can be felt almost immediately. When you abandon the typical slouch or otherwise exaggerated posture to which you are probably accustomed and assume the upright pose we describe here, with the spine fully and easefully extended, you will find that your breathing suddenly and easily becomes full and deep, and you feel alert, strong, and fully alive. That is how you should feel all the time. Appropriate posture simply attunes the physical body to the infinite intensity of universal life through the medium of the etheric energy field or body. Right posture (and all conscious exercise) simply helps to plug you in. It does not involve mystic feats or heroic attainments of any kind.

D. *Consciously establish or generate the present position of the body from the center of gravity in the region of the navel.* The specific center of gravity, or apex of the great vital center of the human body, is a point approximately three fingers' width below and behind the umbilical scar. This seat of the vital center is on the same horizontal axis as the skeletal conjunction of the spine and pelvis.

Traditional cultures have valued the great region of the navel as the seat of life, of physical, moral, and even spiritual force. In a strong, sane, and upright man or woman, the navel center is full of life-force. Such a one moves naturally in the earthly world from this life-center. He does not habitually strain or weaken the physical body, or dissipate life-energy by moving as if the center of gravity were in the legs, the lower abdomen, or the chest. Such movement would be mechanically unlawful. Its consequences are backaches, tension, muscle strains, shortness of breath, and the like, as well as emotional and psychological distress.

The appropriate, lawful, graceful, economic way to make any physical movement is to maintain the upper body in the fundamental posture we have described here, and to move, via the hips, from the center of gravity in the lower navel region.

Probably the simplest way to adapt to the basic posture is to learn it in the standing position, and then adapt it to other activities. There is only one other essential point to be made about the standing posture:

E. *When you stand still, distribute the weight of the physical body on both feet, centering on the ball*

*or broad part of each foot, rather than the heel, and
slightly to the outside.* The heel and the back part of
the foot should be used to balance the body, not to
support its weight. If you could hang a plumb line
from a point directly above the head through the
body, it would fall to the broadest part of the foot,
not to the heel. This imaginary plumb line indicates
the natural vertical alignment of the body.

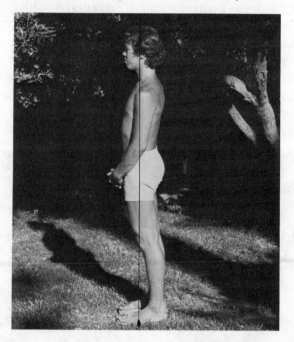

To test your stance and the distribution of body
weight on your feet, try this test: Raise your heels off
the floor without shifting or adjusting your body. If
you have to lean forward before your heels can rise
from the floor, then the weight of your body is in-
correctly distributed. When the weight of the body is
correctly supported by the front, wide part of the foot
(with most of the pressure falling slightly toward the
outside edge of the foot), you will not have to move the
body forward in order to lift your heels off the floor.

Sitting

When sitting, apply the same basic principles as when standing. Tuck the buttocks directly under the trunk, rather than allowing them to protrude behind, and maintain the "flattened" lower back and erect, slightly stretched spine and neck. In this position, the pelvic "bowl" remains upright and balanced, and the weight of the body hangs from the spine and rests directly on the buttocks and upper thighs, which form a firm base for sitting. The body's center of gravity is thus maintained in the navel region. When you have to move from side to side while sitting, lean with the whole upper part of the torso, minimizing the degree to which you curve and bend the spine and neck, and keeping the lower body stable. When you lean forward, lean at the hips.

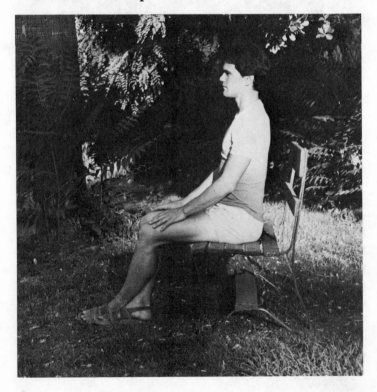

Walking and Moving

A. *The appropriate, lawful, graceful, economic, and strong way to walk, or enter into any vertical physical movement, is to establish the upper and lower portions of the body in the fundamental posture we have described, and to move, via the hips, from the center of gravity, or the vital center, in the lower navel region.*

B. *When you walk, hold the body in the natural erect posture, keep the hips flexible, and move them alternately forward and back, not from side to side, lifting each hip slightly at the beginning of each stride.*

C. *With each stride, extend the leg fully with the knee straight, and allow the foot to assume a right angle to the leg so that the heel makes first contact with the ground.* Just before the left leg lifts for a stride, the body is pushed forward by that leg, and the weight of the body passes from the heel to the ball of the right foot. As the left leg lifts and moves forward, the right leg is straightened at the knee, and then it pushes the body forward in turn and begins to lift for its own stride.

D. *As you walk, hold the head high, the chest up, and the upper torso erect and relaxed. Look directly forward along the horizontal median, neither up into the air nor down to the ground at your feet.* Walking with a slouch, or with eyes to the ground, reinforces subjective inwardness and reflection. In contrast, this natural discipline opens the body and brings energy and attention into the field of relations.

Walking is an excellent form of exercise when done in this way, with a strong stride that uses the whole body without strain, not just the legs. The key to walking properly, as with all other bodily action, is to move from the hips so that the center of gravity is maintained in the vital center. If you do this, it will be natural to hold the head and upper torso in their upright and relaxed positions. Walking with a firm, lengthy stride engages not only all the hip and leg muscles, but the muscles of the stomach, the back, the shoulders, chest, and arms. Breathe deeply when you walk, in easy rhythm with your stride, in the natural way we describe later in this chapter, in the section entitled "Consciously Breathe the Energy of Life."

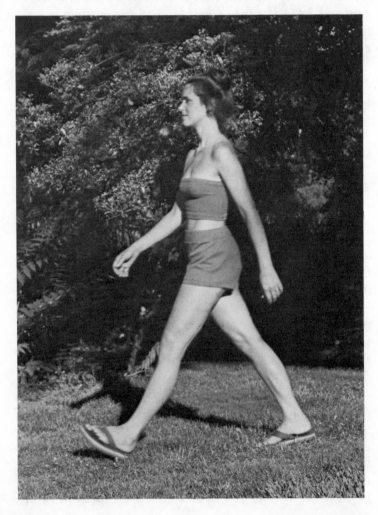

E. *When moving from a vertical position toward the horizontal and below, to perform an action such as lifting, do not bend from the waist, but move into a squatting or nearly squatting position, in which the back remains straight, and rise or lift with the power of the legs, rather than straining the back. But when moving the body from the vertical toward the horizontal and below, and no act of lifting external weight is involved, then bending, rotating, and moving from the waist are usually both graceful and mechanically appropriate, as long as the back is kept essentially straight.*

The Key to Correct Posture

The key to correct posture of the body, whether you are standing, sitting, walking, or performing complex actions, is that the muscular or soft parts of the body must rest on the skeletal structure, chiefly the pelvis and the spine. When the body is properly aligned, you should be able to stand and sit for long periods without shifting the body and without experiencing aching muscles. When your muscles become painful after you have been sitting or standing for a time, it is a sign of undue stress, an indication that the muscles are being tensed, or used by themselves to support the body weight.

Practice the correct posture by standing, sitting, walking, and moving as we have indicated here. Observe how you continually have to adjust the body until you become familiar with these essentially easy and natural postures and forms of action. You will probably experience some difficulty, not merely physical but also psychological and emotional, in adapting to these correct postures (and in learning how to breathe properly while maintaining them). These postural exercises gradually accomplish, through applied personal responsibility and adaptation, what is abruptly and externally effected through such therapeutic methods as structural integration, and other forms of body manipulation, which often trigger sudden intense psychological-emotional releases and traumas as areas of chronic psycho-physical contraction are broken down.[1] The same catharsis or purging may occur through these simple exercises, though probably not in such a dramatic form. Simply recognize all psychological and emotional difficulties as signs of purification and re-adaptation of the body-being, and proceed with your practice.

Consciously Breathe the Energy of Life

You can easily see that you do not create the process of breathing, any more than you create the lungs. Nor do you have the power to stop it and still maintain the consciousness that willed it to stop. Actually, you are *being breathed,* as you may come to realize after practicing conscious exercise for a while.

Bubba Free John has said of this:

> The process of breathing arises simulta-
> neously with the physical body, as does the
> sense of separate identity by which the whole
> body integrates its many functions. It is not
> that breathing is created and controlled by

---

1. This is not to discourage the appropriate and timely use of professional therapeutic approaches to bodily reintegration, such as structural integration (or "Rolfing"), chiropractic, polarity therapy, and various Oriental and Western forms of massage. You may, on occasion, find one or more of these therapies quite beneficial. Before taking any treatment, however, you should understand and become essentially proficient in the personal and responsible disciplines of posture, breathing, and conscious action communicated in *Conscious Exercise and the Transcendental Sun.* Once you are strong and disciplined bodily in this way, you will be better able to maintain the structural realignments effected by therapeutic work.

an other (or Other) outside. It is simply that our consciousness cannot be radically differentiated from the process of life and breath. Breathing is a cycle at infinity. It is not created and controlled by any "one." It is a pattern within an infinite pattern of relations.

Therefore, it is only appropriate to participate consciously and directly, with feeling, free of subjective conceptualizing and imagining, in the cosmic energy process that is manifesting as the body and the whole universe in every moment. Simply breathe, and feel it. Feel that you are receiving conscious, revitalizing, and transforming life-energy when you inhale, and that you are releasing accumulated tensions, toxins, and negative psychological and emotional conditions when you exhale.

There is a right way to breathe during conscious exercise. Practice breathing this way as you read the following description of the mechanics of the life-breath.

A. *Breathe via the nose, with the mouth closed.*

B. *Initiate the breath from the heart (the conscious, feeling, psychic core of the body-being)—that is, initiate the breath with the power of emotion, or whole body feeling—through and with the throat, to the navel.*

C. *When you inhale, draw in, relax into, and conduct the life-energy of the universe with the whole being, even through the entire skin surface of the whole physical body, head to toe, down or into the vital center, the great life region, whose felt center is behind and below the umbilical scar.* Feel the life-energy at and from this life center, radiating through the whole being as fullness.

D. *Inhale fully, with deep feeling of heart and*

body, completely filling the lungs with air and the whole body with life-force. As the life-force moves through the body with the inhalation, it is first sensed in the soft-life region of the solar plexus. As it is drawn downward, it fills and expands the lower body, even the genitals and then the legs and feet. You may also feel a slight tingling sensation at the perineum, which is the lowest or terminal point in the etheric "pathway" of the body-being. Then the chest and upper regions of the body open, including the neck and head, and the entire body from the crown to the perineum, even to the toes, is tangibly permeated with vibrant energy.

E. *When you exhale, do not discard the energy itself or allow it to dissipate, but release and relax all hold on it, allowing it to radiate, from the vital center and the whole body. Allow and feel the pleasurable force of life to be pumped by the heart through the entire body (the limbs, the belly, the sex organs, the head, the teeth and hair and nails, etc.) and the universe. Exhale fully, and with deep feeling of heart and body. Let the energy pervade the whole body and the universe to infinity, and release, via that radiating and expansive energy, all accumulated conditions, positive or negative, so that inhalation may bring what is new and thus become an instrument of change and refreshment.*

To become adept at right breathing will require, in most cases, careful and constant practice. You may, for instance, have some difficulty inhaling *through and with the fully open and relaxed throat.* Until the process becomes natural to you, follow this procedure randomly to feel the difference between the right and wrong ways of breathing: First breathe in an exaggerated fashion with the nose, sniffing deeply, even audibly, through the nostrils. Then relax the whole area of the nose and mouth completely. Let the tongue curve forward and up, resting lightly against the hard palate. And rest your attention at the rear and the base of the throat. Now let the muscles of this area open and become the channel of inhalation. Allow the facial muscles around the nose and mouth to remain at rest as you breathe deeply, with feeling and from the heart, and make an audible "drawing" sound as the breath passes through the throat, passing down its back side.

You should notice a pronounced difference between these two forms of breathing. By tendency, you breathe in the unnatural way, from and with the nose or the mouth. As you engage the practice of appropriate breathing, you will observe randomly that the mechanisms by which the body opens to the breath and the life-force tend to remain obstructed or else to open only partially and awkwardly when you breathe unnaturally. But you will find that the entire gross bodily being, both elemental and etheric, opens spontaneously or effortlessly when the breath and life-force are conducted in the natural way, via the throat, with feeling, from the heart, to the vital center.

Clearly, it is not air that is being drawn into the navel and lower regions of the body, but life-force, energy, "prana," or "spirit." Physical air and the process of biochemical respiration in the lungs constitute only secondary, grosser aspects of the dynamics of the breath. Breathing is principally a spiritual process. That is, it principally and directly involves the higher physics of the etheric or pranic body, and only secondarily involves the elemental or physical being. Thus, it is also natural, especially as practice matures, to feel the "in-spiration" or reception of life-energy, not only through the valve of the throat, but through the entire skin surface of the physical body. When the breath is felt in this way, the conscious being is beginning to include direct perception and enjoyment of the subtlest of the gross elements, which is ether or life-energy, along with its perception and utilization of the denser elements, which are earth, water, fire, and air.

During common activities, breathe easily, but fully and deeply, and coordinate the breath in a natural (not self-conscious) rhythm with alterations of posture and other bodily movements. Let the vital center, below and behind the navel, receive, enjoy, release, and distribute every cycle of the life-breath. When the breath is full, you will spontaneously enjoy a relaxation of all fixed or obsessive mentality and emotional reactivity, and you will sense an opening in the mind and the emotions as well as in the living body. (For more discussion of right breathing, see chapter four, "The Weather System of the Life Sun: Pranayama, the Control of Life in Breath.")

Summary Points to Remember

Body

This is the key to correct posture: The weight of the soft parts of the body should rest naturally on the large, structural bones, especially the spine and pelvis.

These are the signs of the fundamental human posture (under the conditions of the natural, waking state):

☐ The upper body is firmly erect, with the chest held high, the neck and spine simultaneously stretched and relaxed, and the face and eyes facing directly forward (not downward and polarized to the earth, nor upward, polarized to the sky of mind).

☐ The head rests directly on the spine, and the weight of the body hangs or extends from the spine, the vertical axis.

☐ The pelvis, the horizontal axis, is brought forward and up, perpendicular to the spine, so that the small of the back is nearly flattened.

☐ When you are standing, the weight of the body should rest on the broad parts of the feet, and slightly to the outside, rather than on the heels.

☐ When you are sitting, the buttocks should be tucked under the upper body.

☐ When you are walking, the hips should move forward and back, rather than side to side, lifting slightly at the beginning of each stride, and the heel should make the first contact with the ground.

Breath

☐ Receive and relax with full feeling into limit-less life-energy with each inhalation, and release-relax all accumulated, contracted, and negative conditions of the being with each exhalation, allowing the energy to permeate the entire body-being and the universe.

☐ Breathe with feeling from the heart, via the throat, and to the vital center, the great life region, below and behind the navel.

Mind

☐ Let the mind be present as full feeling-attention of the whole body and its relations rather than obsessive thinking and imagining in the head. Thus, direct every functional activity with free and natural feeling-attention and feeling-intention, as a form of conscious exercise, following and coordinating the integration of the physical body (form) and the etheric body (energy and breath).

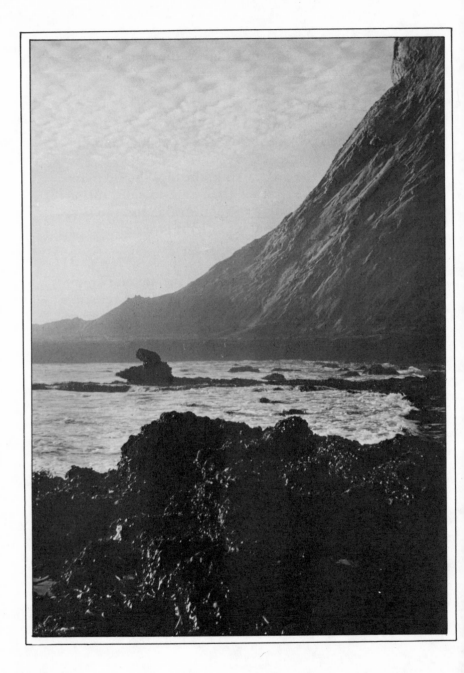

3

The Routines of Formal Exercise

You want to manipulate your subjectivity—your feelings, your thinking, your conceptions, and your feeling-conceptions. You want to change them before you will change your way of life. You want to be free inside before you will love, before you act differently. You must act differently first, and not be concerned that the feeling and thinking aspect of the being remains full of tendencies. You must not be concerned about them. They are just the signs of the old way of living. You must act in love, in radiance, with energy, with life, in all your relations, in your disposition moment to moment, under all conditions. You will observe in the midst of such action that the subjective dimension is also gradually penetrated and transformed. Its negativity, its reactivity, becomes unnecessary and ultimately obsolete by virtue of your different action.

Stop presuming the separate position. Stop being angry and sorrowful and fearful in your relations and bring energy into them. Be happy in them. Be enthusiastic in them. Bring life to all beings. Bring life to the tree. Bring life to the doorknob and to me! And you will see your subjective life changing, over time. It may remain completely wretched for 25,000 births. Do not be concerned about it. Act differently on the basis of what you have heard.

Bubba Free John
The Paradox of Instruction

3

Bubba Free John has adapted the formal routines described in the following pages from the traditional systems of Calisthenics and Hatha Yoga. Calisthenics vigorously exercise the cardio-vascular system through fast movement and rhythmic contraction and relaxation of the muscles. We recommend that you perform them in the morning (after study or meditation, if you are engaged in religious or spiritual practice, and before breakfast), to invigorate and enliven the body. Such brisk exercise in the morning fully adapts the living being to the waking and bodily conditions that will prevail during the day.

In contrast, Hatha Yoga exercises are subtler activities, in which physical movements are secondary to fixed poses and the breathing of life-energy. Hatha Yoga relaxes and harmonizes the body. It is therefore recommended for either the evening or the end of the working day (at least a half-hour before or an hour after the evening meal). This calming exercise at the end of the day provides a refreshing break in the routine of activities, whether you have been sedentary or active. You can perform Hatha Yoga with equal benefit and enjoyment an hour or so before sleep, if you cannot make time earlier.

Surya Namaskar is a combination of action and

postures, a harmony of Calisthenics and Hatha Yoga. It can be practiced either as a Calisthenic, with energetic movements and breathing, or as a slow and rhythmic sequence of Hatha Yoga poses, in which you relax briefly into each position before assuming the next. You should perform the Surya Namaskar several times in succession before each routine of formal exercise, morning and evening, to loosen and oxygenate the entire body.

The Principles of "Conscious Exercise," to Be Applied to Surya Namaskar, Calisthenics, and Hatha Yoga, by Bubba Free John

Physical exercises or poses, whether those described in this book or obtained from other sources, are not in themselves forms of "conscious exercise." "Conscious exercise" is a point of view relative to our application to exercise and to common activities. The physical exercises and poses you adapt to your daily formal routines are, in themselves, only models for physical movement. Like all ordinary actions, they do not necessarily or inherently require or signify a simultaneous discipline of mind, or attention, or feeling and emotion, or even intentional breathing.

Both physical exercise and ordinary activity, including motionless poses and sedentary occupations, become "conscious exercise" only when they involve the simultaneous and coordinated discipline of mind, emotion, and body in the single medium or environment that is the universal life-force. And only "conscious exercise" may thus be said to be truly human activity, since only when so coordinated are all the conventionally human functions operative and made a single condition of conscious existence.

Practical Guidelines for Performance
of Formal Exercise Routines

1. Perform all exercises in the manner described in chapter one, particularly in the section entitled "The Principles in Action to Which All Exercise and Even Ordinary Activity Must Be Adapted" (p. 35). Coordinate free attention, through full and deep feeling, with cycles of breathing, posture, and action, and thus live in the environment of energy or Light or Love.

2. Bathing and proper scheduling should be associated with formal exercise routines. Upon arising in the morning, it is recommended that you follow this schedule: Brush your teeth and wash or sponge your face, hands, and perhaps the navel region; meditate or study (if you are involved in a religious or spiritual practice of life); perform the Calisthenics routine, preceded by Surya Namaskar; take a shower, alternating hot and cold water; give yourself a dry brush or rough towel massage; and then have breakfast.

Hot and cold alternating showers and baths help keep the body healthy by using the principle of fever to combat disease and stimulate the nervous system. The dry brush or rough towel massage, either before or after showering, helps the body to eliminate toxins released through the skin by allowing the pores to breathe, and rids the body of dead skin cells accumulated during the day and during sleep. It is also suggested that you shower and dry brush either before or after the afternoon or evening Hatha Yoga routine. And be certain that Hatha Yoga is performed at least half an hour before or an hour after the evening meal, since both the taking and the digestion of food require a particular kind of participation of body and life.

3. *Generally, exercise alone, so that you are neither distracted nor inhibited by the presence of another.*

4. *Set aside time twice each day when you can exercise without interruption and without the pressure of other obligations.*

5. *Never miss an exercise session, and exercise for at least ten minutes without breaking the routine on each occasion.*

6. *Whenever possible, exercise out of doors (in the sun if possible, but don't get overheated), or at least near a source of fresh air, such as an open window or door.* In areas where polluted air prevails, it is better to exercise inside with doors and windows closed.

7. *Wear minimal and loose-fitting clothing whenever you exercise.*

8. *Use a mat of natural, non-synthetic materials, neither too hard nor too soft, for performing each of these routines.*

9. *You should develop a systematic way to exercise, flowing from one exercise or pose to the next.* Each of the routines in this chapter has been arranged in a sequence that serves such a natural, balanced flow of movement and posture. Even the Calisthenics should be practiced as a step-by-step routine, with no variation of order from day to day, in the same continuous fashion as Surya Namaskar and Hatha Yoga.

10. *Avoid exercising violently or beyond the level of your endurance,* as strain only develops or traps toxins in the body and depletes the strength of the nervous system. Never exercise to the point of exhaustion. Formal exercise should be enjoyable and refreshing! It should not obstruct energy or dissipate your vital force. Where there are no physical, emotional, mental, or psychic obstructions, and the physical is naturally attuned to the etheric being and

the universal life-energy, the force of life is effectively limitless.

In formal exercise, be certain to apply the same foundation disciplines of attention, breath and energy, and physical form that you have already adapted to the ordinary or non-formal actions of life, such as standing and walking.

11. *Always rest after practicing the exercise routines.* Follow every formal session of conscious exercise with at least 3-4 minutes of rest, in which the body, breath, and mind are harmonized and thoroughly relaxed. (See the "Dead Pose" on page 132 for instructions on how to rest consciously.)

If you are busy or hurried, you may feel an urge to move directly from the exercise routines back into daily activities without resting. Do not yield to that inclination. The rest period is as necessary a part of any formal routine as the movements themselves. Without rest, your exercises may only create a subtly inharmonious condition that is both physically and psychically disturbing.

12. *Develop a rhythmic, interested, life-supporting routine of life.* The character of your activity in any moment should be simple or straightforward, full of feeling and livingness — but the pattern of every day and every significant period of time should be a complex of changes or interests, a rhythmic movement through the many aspects of action and repose, relationship and transcendence. Right diet and work, responsible sexual intimacy, true study and service, and right Communion with the Condition of all conditions are all essential to human sanity, and peace among us.

Exercise According to Your Capacity and Increase Your Proficiency by Degrees

The exercises in this book are not difficult or complicated. If you enjoy good health and are not disabled, you should be able to perform most of them adequately, if not perfectly, from the beginning of your practice. But you may find that a period of adjustment is necessary before you can perform certain of the exercises with correct coordination of movement, breath, and posture. For instance, if you have tight, constricted muscles and tendons in the back and the legs, you may have difficulty assuming certain of the Surya Namaskar or Hatha Yoga poses.

Therefore, *at the beginning, you should modify the routines according to your capacity, and then work toward perfecting them over time.* The modifications you make may even be permanent, as long as they serve rather than undermine your participation in conscious exercise as a discipline. *Increase your proficiency by degrees, without straining, free of the impulse to "force" the body unnaturally into the perfect performance of the exercises.*

Pregnant women should be careful not to exercise violently. Generally, they should not practice the formal routines at all beyond the first month or two of pregnancy. They should, however, be mindful of posture, since the body tends during pregnancy to compensate for the weight of the fetus by adapting to improper posture. Pregnant women should therefore use the postural disciplines, in coordination with the breath, as the daily exercise "routine."

In general, every individual should observe these postural disciplines *as exercise* under all conditions, all day long—and especially if, for some urgent reason, you have no choice but to skip part of your regular daily routine. Those who have bodily mal-functions that prevent their performing the exercise routines should use the postural disciplines as exercise more or less exclusively.

(As with any practice related to the health of the body, it is advisable for all to consult a physician, particularly one trained in naturopathic medicine, before beginning any program of exercise.)

When You Are Proficient

When you have learned the basic routines well, you should feel free to modify and add to them. Other Calisthenic exercises and Hatha Yoga poses may be found in the many books on these subjects, and you should also feel free to add dance movements, extended walks, jogging, "roving" (a random combination of walking and running), conscious and deliberate participation in sports and games, and the like. Also, certain appliances, such as the slant board, the bicycle (stationary or mobile), and other devices that are combined with Isometrics and/or Calisthenics may be utilized as extensions of the Calisthenics routine. *You may also wish to perform Calisthenics or Hatha Yoga exercises in a different order from that pre-scribed in the following pages.* Feel free to do so, but always be sure to maintain the principle of the sequences offered in this book, which maintains a rhythmic balance of contractive-tensing and expansive-stretching exercises that work on the same parts of the body.

Once you are proficient, beyond laziness, and sensi-tive to your own bodily tendencies, beyond self-indulgence, you may vary your practice. Most people should continue to exercise vigorously and formally, to the point of breaking into a sweat, at least once every other day. Some require this on a daily basis. Others should exercise in this manner even more frequently or for more prolonged periods.

Everyone should apply themselves, either at fixed times or randomly, but daily, to various Hatha Yoga poses, stretching exercises, light application of Surya Namaskar, and so forth. And, of course, the basic approach of "conscious exercise" should be applied to all common activities as long as we live.

Conscious Exercise and the Transcendental Sun is not intended to be an exhaustive description of any of the systems of exercise recommended. Rather, it is a general guide to the affair of conscious exercise, to be applied under all conditions and in relation to any or all systems of formal exercise. For detailed considerations of the exercise systems themselves, you should read and consult good source texts. (See the list of recommended books at the end of the present volume.)

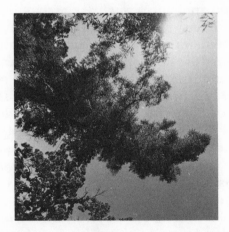

The Internal "Locks" of the Whole Body, by Bubba Free John

The living human body is a system or structure for the conduction of life. The physical body is contacted by or unified with mind, or attention, via the pervading medium of life-force. The present capacity of the complex of attention, feeling, and bodily form to conduct the life-power is its general state of responsibility, or "conductivity."

The same life-force pervades both the physical body and its environment. The physical body does not "contain," or grasp and hold, the life-force, but simply communes or communicates with the all-pervading life-force, or manifest light, and intensifies the sense and effect of the life-force through feeling, or psycho-physical emotion. Attention (including intention and controlled thought) and the control of posture and activity are the outer limbs or extremities, the opposite poles of the process of living. The center, root, and living core of the process is the life-force or universal energy, apparently cycled through the phases of the breath, but constantly and priorly communicated in, as, and through us via the process of feeling.

Feeling is either obstructed and reactive or unobstructed and non-reactive. Reactive emotions, such as fear, sorrow, and anger, are forms of recoil. They contract the mechanisms of the whole body, and obstruct or attenuate the conductivity, and thus the responsibility, of the whole being. When there is simple, direct, and native participation in the state of life, there is no reactivity, but a pleasurable, relational force and radiance. This is love, or unobstructed conductivity. In that case, the responsibility of the whole body-being is optimum, and Communion with the Real Condition or Truth of all conditions is possible, and even native to that instant.

The cycle of breathing is a reflection of the present state of conductivity, and thus responsibility, of the individual. Indeed, the cycle of breathing, or conductivity of life, is senior to all subjectivity, all reactivity. Breath and emotion are identical. We feel and breathe simultaneously, as a single event. Unobstructed feeling, or love, is senior to the physiological action of the breath, but simultaneous with it. Love is creative or causative relative to breath and life.

Reactive feeling, or negative and caused emotions, are secondary to the physiological action of the breath. Shocks of life modify the breath-life pattern directly, and create contracted emotional patterns, as well as the sense that love and good feelings depend on reasons or circumstantial stimulation. Thus, by experience and reaction, our native responsibility for love in every moment is weakened. Shocks of life and breath are creative or causative relative to reactive or obstructed emotions.

The creative task of the living being is to remain responsible for its native disposition and conductivity, even through and in the midst of the shocks and impositions of experience. It is the Law of Sacrifice or Love that is hidden in every breath. If we abide as love, with free attention in all action, then we remain in the creative or responsible position relative to life, breath, action, and Realization. But if we abide in our subjectivity, self-possessed, distracted — by the obsessive sound of thinking—from feeling in the infinite pattern of relations, then we are irresponsible, subject to random experience, unable to conduct life, or to breathe openly, or to act sanely and humanly, or to Realize Truth.

The feeling cycle of the breath is thus the center of life and all our relations. The conscious feeling of the bodily and relational cycle of breath and life, under conditions of action and repose, is central to our well-being, our good relations, and to the whole affair of conscious exercise. Therefore, it is essential to realize the critical factors and events in the feeling cycle of breathing.

The physical body is always already fully permeated by all-pervading energy, or life-force. It never becomes empty or filled, but it is only either more or less directly and presently in a condition of communication or communion with the universal life. We fluctuate or "phase" in our state of feeling moment to moment. We also chronically feel reactive or contracted and negative emotional conditions, from fear and sorrow and anger to relatively modest anxiety and sadness and despair to depression and dullness and boredom. Therefore, we are also chronically tending toward a condition of non-communication of life or energy on the basis of the effects of experience or reactions to experience in every moment.

The only way to realize a present degree of maximum intensity, communicated in, as, and through the whole body-being, is to feel without obstruction or contraction. Then we abide in the native intensity of the universally present energy, life, or light. That feeling is named "love" and "sacrifice," or "surrender." It is the unqualified feeling and the native intensity of the whole body-being that characterizes us when we simply look and feel and are and act completely happy. In our chronic condition, we tend to manifest such happiness or love—in other words, we tend to communicate or commune with the native force of existence—only when events *cause* us to react with complete, unobstructed feeling. Thus, only in the rare moments of good fortune or fulfillment, the moments equivalent to suddenly getting a gift of a million dollars, do we consent to feel and to exist as our native intensity.

This is the chronic problem of man—that he does not consent to feel as he *is* but only as he is caused to feel. We feel according to our present circumstances rather than our prior or native intensity. The spiritual obligation of every man or woman is to realize the prior intensity of life in every moment. And this is possible only if there is true, present, and radical "hearing" of the argument of Truth and of life itself. Only then will we consent or even be able to look and feel and be and act completely happy under all conditions.

The discipline of "conscious exercise" is a part of the whole spiritual discipline that obliges devotees in the Way of Divine Ignorance. All others may also apply at least this part of the wisdom of the whole body, and so benefit all of us by becoming more stable, healthy, and responsible for life and feeling.

And feeling, as you see, is the key to the functional wisdom of the whole body. Feeling unlocks the contractions of the reactive body life, and permits a free communication between attention and action. Once we enjoy such self-control, which moves us positively into the pattern of relations, other so-called "locks" may usefully be added to the feeling control of the body.

In the simplest terms, the living body is an expression of two tendencies, uses, or currents of life. And, again in the simplest or most basic terms, these tendencies are the two motions of contraction and expansion, or reception and release. There is a negative or exclusive and unbalanced expression of each of these tendencies. When reactivity, or reaction to experience, becomes stronger than the force of life and unobstructed or free feeling-attention that we commonly bring to experience, then reception and contraction disable us. We become self-possessed, confined to subjectivity, negatively emotional, vitally weak, and self-defeating in action. Then expansion or release is confined to patterns of mere self-indulgence, so that we are constantly emptied until death.

But there is a positive or true functional development of each of these motions, when they are in balance, and when attention and bodily form and action are controlled by full central communion or feeling into the universal environment of the life-force. In that case, even each breath becomes a balanced cycle of reception-release, contraction-expansion, in the constant field of fully felt intensity or life.

It has already been considered how the inhalation of breath, or life, is associated with reception, infilling, and natural conductivity or movement toward the whole body. Likewise, the exhalation is associated with release of the wastes, the accumulated contents or old circumstances and adaptations of life (not the release or emptying of life itself), and natural expansion, which is conductivity or movement from the whole body outward. This dual cycle is generated from the heart (the feeling center), and enacted between the apparent entrance of breath at the nose and the vital or abdominal center below. The cycle of breathing moves to and from the vital abdominal center. The vital center is not filled and emptied in the process, but it is rhythmically active as the bodily center wherein the felt intensity of the universal life is constantly and priorly communicated with and expressed.

When we breathe, we should breathe with the sense that the whole body rests or abides always and already in the universal, all-pervading life field. Thus, the vital center and the head are both, equally and always, in perfect and constant contact with the light of life. When the cycle of breathing is generated, it should not be felt that life only enters the nose and then goes down to the vital center, but that the whole body breathes or communes with the universal life. The nose, throat, vital center, and heart are simply mechanisms or parts of the conversation between the whole body and the all-pervading life.

On inhalation, the breath or life is to be felt as if drawn or intensified via the whole surface of the body. Secondarily, it tends also to be felt as if passing down from the nose to the vital center. Therefore, there is a tendency toward the secondary feeling that life is passing down and out through the lower body on inhalation. There is also the sense, at the full point of inhalation, that the breath-force is tending not to be retained at the vital center but, rather, to escape by recoiling upward, through the chest, throat, and nose.

Likewise, on exhalation, the breath or life is to be felt as if expanding as intensity throughout the whole body and through the whole surface of the body to infinity. Secondarily, it tends also to be felt as if it is passing up and out, leaving the vital center and passing out through the nose. Therefore, there is a tendency toward the secondary feeling that life is being taken out from the vital center and dispersed via the upper body on exhalation.

Thus, on both inhalation and exhalation there is a similar and chronic sensation, secondary to the primary process of whole body reception-release. (The primary process is without loss of energy, since energy is all-pervading, and the body does not take it in or out, but simply participates in it with either more or less direct, unobstructed, and full feeling.) The sensation awakened relative to the secondary process is, in each case, the sensation that the life-force is entering and/or leaving the vital center.

If the life-energy can enter or leave the vital center, then the vital center exists, and the whole body feels, as if it were always already empty, dependent on a process that fills it, and subject to a process that empties it.

The conviction of emptiness is demonstrated at the heart, in inhibition of feeling. Fear is the logic of independent or separate and priorly empty existence. And fear is the chronic "feeling" that controls the breath of life.

Therefore, our living and spiritual obligation is to enter fully into the primary process of life. This means we must abide constantly in the sense that the whole body, from the feeling heart, from and to and through the whole surface or skin of the body, and via the vital center, is always already existing in an all-pervading, unqualified, and universal field of energy, life, or light. It is only because the life-force is associated with the incoming and outgoing cycle of the breath that we feel life itself comes and goes, whereas in fact life is constant, and the cycle of breath is only a play of feeling-attention on the universal energy that always already pervades the whole body, the vital center, the heart, and the mind. If feeling can be full and constant, then it is no longer subject to the apparent cycle or "phasing" of the breath. Then our immortal position begins to become clear, at the heart, prior to mind and body. Therefore, we are constantly obliged by the Law of Sacrifice, Love, or Radiance.

The sense of the prior fullness and eternal conservation of life or light may be presumed to be simply or
factually true on the basis of consideration of science
and experience. Thus, anyone may practice "conscious exercise" who has at least minimal sympathy
with the higher evidence of science and life. But the
full or optimum practice depends on prior Realization of the Truth of the whole body, and such
Realization depends on true hearing of the radical
argument of Truth, as communicated by one who
is alive in its Realization. Just so, the practice itself
is a whole life of full devotional practice in the
spiritual Company of such a one and in cooperation
with other devotees.

To continue with this discussion of the secondary
sense of prior emptiness or functional loss of life-
energy, it is because of these secondary tendencies,
or the habitual association with the feeling that the
whole body is empty and emptying, at the vital center
as it breathes, that certain "locks" or contractions of
the feeling body are appropriate to add to formal
exercise and even to random moments of our ordinary
living.

During formal exercise, whenever the inhaled
breath becomes full, or the exhaled breath is complete, it is often appropriate to lock the *breath* into
or out of the body. (Remember, the secondary process
is the breath cycle in itself, and the primary process
is the direct participation in the universally and
priorly communicated life field. The "locks" are
activities relative to the secondary process, or the
breath cycle, and are only intended to reduce the
experiential effects or presumptions of energy loss and
emptiness.) The first of these, the throat lock, is
generally only to be done briefly, and only when the
physical activity permits it. It may be done by pressing
the chin lightly or moderately into the jugular knot at

the base of the throat. If physical movement is intense, then the lock may be performed as a feeling-intention only, or simply a light constriction at the lower throat.

The principal lock of the body, however, is the anus-perineum-genital lock, at the crest of inhalation and in the initiation of exhalation. As the sense of bodily infilling increases during inhalation, the tendency to feel energy passing out through the lower body begins. Thus, as the sense of fullness begins, the anus-perineum-genital area should be lightly or moderately tensed, inwards and upwards. At the point of fullness of inhalation, the throat lock may also be used, when felt to be natural and appropriate. Likewise, particularly in Hatha Yoga routines, the anus-perineum-genital lock may be supplemented by a lock at the navel, performed by lightly or moderately tensing or drawing in at the navel and the upper crown of the abdomen.

As exhalation begins, the throat lock should be released, and the locks of the anus-perineum-genital area and the navel may be lightly or moderately increased, as exhalation continues and the region of the abdomen and solar plexus tends to become concave. And, at the end of exhalation, the exhaled breath may be "held out" briefly by one or the other form of the throat lock.

The anus-perineum-genital lock may be used at random during ordinary activity. It is particularly useful because of the chronic sense and tendency we have of being empty and of emptying the body of its life via the cycle of breathing and through the lower mechanisms or vital functions of the gross life.

Contraction of the anus-perineum-genital area (with or without the other two locks) should not become chronic, as in a case of anxiety, but it should be exercised at random, in association with the inhalation-exhalation cycle, as just described.

At random times, the anus-perineum-genital area may be rhythmically contracted upward and then released, for several moments, slowly or relatively quickly. This tends to counter the downward-outward muscular and nervous system pattern chronically generated via the organs of elimination and generation.

These locks are natural forms of control of the physical body and the nervous system in association with breathing, or the sense of relative emptiness or fullness of bodily energy. You should adapt them yourself to the inhalation-exhalation pattern of formal conscious exercise, including sedentary "pranayama," and to random moments of ordinary life. The locks are a secondary practice, to be used when and if you will. The primary practice is the simple one of reception-release in whole body feeling. The locks only serve to counter some of the secondary side effects or accompaniments of the feeling cycle of the breath, wherein it is felt that energy is being channeled and lost through a single area of the body, rather than expressed constantly and radiantly via the whole body. The primary practice is the present and radical return to unobstructed and full feeling, which is love, or Radiance, and breathing from the prior position of unqualified Life or Fullness. (Prior to initiation or true Realization of this Fullness as Divine Presence or Reality, you should simply exercise and breathe with full, whole body feeling rather than merely mental intention.)

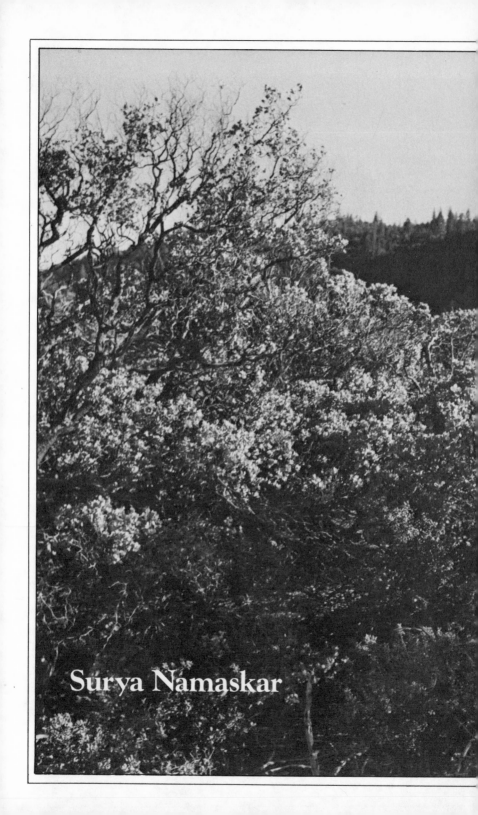

Surya Namaskar

e feeling that the breath is moving alternately
side. The effect of this way of breathing in
Namaskar is to balance and harmonize the
ons of the two sides of the body and nervous
(See chapter four, "The Weather System of
e Sun: Pranayama, the Control of Life in
," for more discussion of the balancing of the
d energies of the body-being.)
u choose, you may do Surya Namaskar in both
lternately or at random, perhaps using the
m of breathing in the morning, with Calis-
, and the alternating form in the evening, with
Yoga. Or, if the alternate method is not com-
e or natural to you, you may choose to use the
basic method exclusively.
a Namaskar, as traditionally practiced, is part
whole routine of Hatha Yoga exercises. In
times, and even to this day, many practi-
have made it a literal "sun prayer," looking
e sun, directly or indirectly, while they move
n the cycle of poses. The purpose of such prac-
o allow the direct force of sunlight to awaken
ensify the glands and subtle centers of energy
ht in the midbrain and other regions of the
lthough our practice of Surya Namaskar has
mystical purpose, Bubba does recommend
henever possible, we face the sun while doing
ctice, and allow its light to fall directly or at
liquely into the eyes at random moments. The
for this is simple and practical: In small quan-
r in greater quantities, if the eyes are properly
l over time) direct sunlight stimulates, heals,
enerates the eyes and, through the eyes, the
lso. Bubba also suggests that Surya Namaskar
done outdoors, in the morning and in the late
on, when the sun is only partially above the

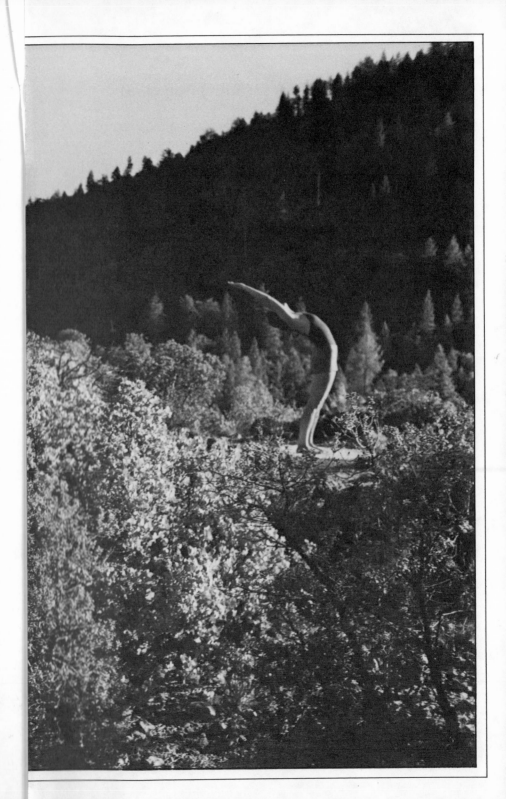

Surya Namaskar (Sun Salutation)

Surya Namaskar is a simple twelve-step exercise routine that uses all the basic muscles and structural relationships of the body. Although it is an apparently simple routine, it is very difficult to perfect, primarily because the body always tends to compensate or adjust itself arbitrarily relative to certain positions. But in the perfection of Surya Namaskar, once you learn the correct form and rhythm, there should be no compensating by any part of the body. The hands and feet should remain in their correct positions in each of the twelve positions. For this reason, do not move from one spot to another when practicing Surya Namaskar, but keep the body confined to the same general space throughout. To aid you in performing the exercise correctly, you may find it helpful to use a small "target" mat for appropriate positioning of the toes and wrists (as shown in the accompanying photograph).

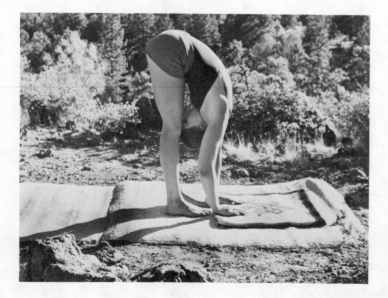

When performing Surya N
as a Calisthenic in the mo
impossible to achieve the pe
at least at first, due to stiffne
concerned, but simply perfor
you can without straining y
form it slowly, as a Hatha
relax briefly in each of the t
allow the body to go limp.
perfect form of each pose, an
always perform the exercises
the sense that you are receivin
and all of the rest of the disci
"conscious exercise."

Try to develop your practic
mum of 5-10 cycles of Surya
basic morning and evening
Namaskar it is best to rest b
before going on to the Hatha
also find a brief rest period
between Surya Namaskar and

There are two variations in
ing during Surya Namaskar
commonly used way is simply t
both nostrils simultaneously,
general description of the b
chapter two. The second way is
nostrils alternately, by simply
side and then the other. Thus,
that you are breathing thro
only, and then exhale with th
breathing through the left no
breath, reverse the cycle—inh
exhaling through the right. A
breath. Do not use any mecha
fingers, to effect this alternate
concentrate on the two nostrils

with t
in eac
Surya
opera
system
the L
Breat
sides

If y
ways,
first
theni
Hath
forta
first

Su
of th
ancie
tione
into
thro
tice
and
and
head
no s
that
this
leas
reas
titie
ada
and
bra
may
afte

horizon. The angle of refraction at such a time heightens the vital energy communicated horizontally, or at eye level, through the sunlight. (It is also good, for this reason, to do this exercise with very little clothing, allowing the rays of the sun to nourish the whole body directly with energy.)

Position 1

A. Stand erect with the feet spread 4-6 inches apart.

B. Relax the whole body, bringing the palms firmly together at the chest.

C. Then inhale, be full, and tense the whole body.

D. Fix the eyes at a generalized point straight ahead (just beneath the physical sun, if possible) with the feeling that you are gazing into an all-pervasive field of light and energy. The whole cycle of Surya Namaskar should be done with the sense of this all-pervading source of light, even if you are indoors, or if you are exercising in the evening after the physical sun has set.

Breathe to the vital center, with the feeling that the pervasive light is its constant source of energy and life.

Relax the eyes, direct your gaze forward, and *feel* the sun-source to be omnipresent, everywhere, not concentrated in any point or object.

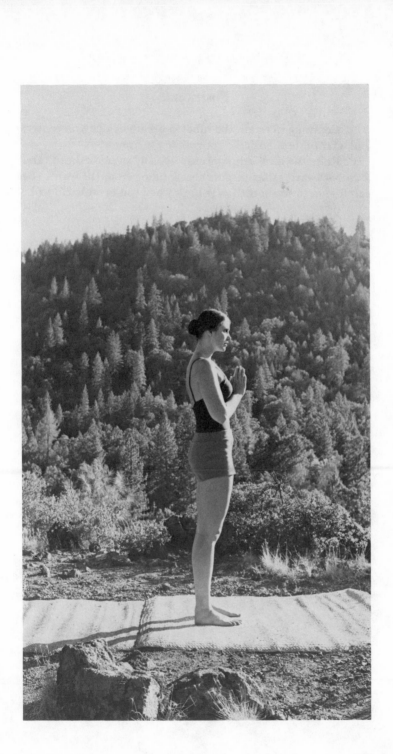

Position 2

A. Continue to retain the inhaled breath at the vital center, and relax the tension of the body while you stretch.

B. Raise the arms straight out, up, and over the head, and arch backward as far as possible, bending from the waist. (Be careful not to strain the lower back when you bend backward.)

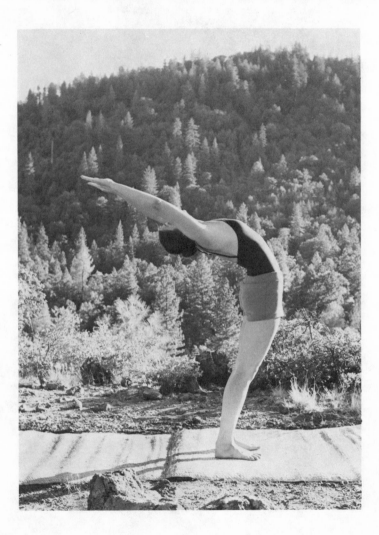

Position 3

A. Exhale and release, thrusting your body forward at the waist, placing the palms down to the outside of the feet, fingers pointing forward.

B. The wrists are directly in line with the big toes. The head is down with the face pressing to the knees. The eyes look toward the stomach and above. Keep the knees straight, but not locked.

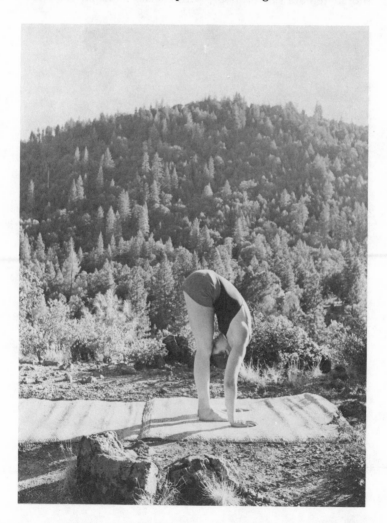

Position 4

A. Inhale as you stretch the left leg back, allowing the knee to touch the floor, and arch the head backward with the eyes looking high above and the hands remaining flat on the floor.

B. The right shin is perpendicular to the floor, pressing the top of the right thigh firmly into the chest. The right foot should remain on the floor, with the heel flat on the floor.

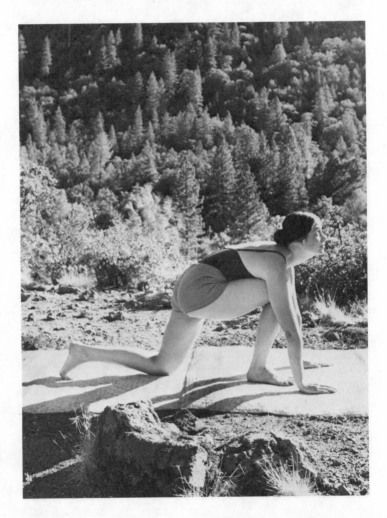

Position 5

A. Retaining the breath, place the right leg back, putting the feet together.

B. At the same time, bend the head down directly in line with the arms.

Keep the legs straight and the heels flat on the floor. This position forms a perfect pyramid or jackknife.

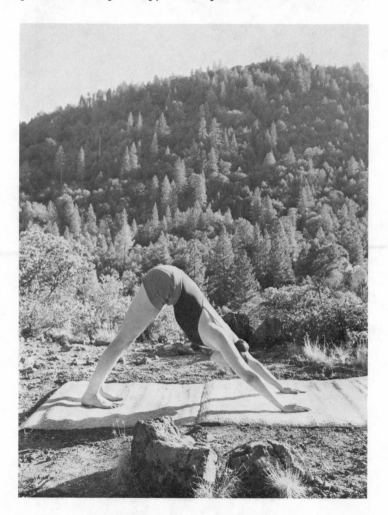

Position 6

A. Without moving the hands and feet, exhale, lowering the body to the floor. Keep the body straight.

B. Keeping the breath exhaled and lying flat on the stomach, arch the back and bring the buttocks into the air, lifting the thighs off the ground. The forehead, chest, and knees are on the ground, and the arms are bent.

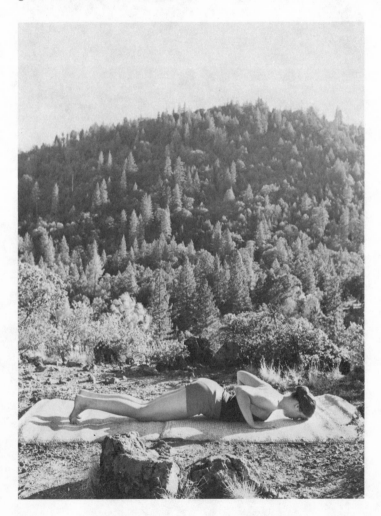

Position 7

A. Inhaling, raise the head and arch the back, bringing the chest and upper stomach region off the floor.

B. The head should be bent back as far as possible, with the eyes looking above and the arms straight. The body is supported by the lower pelvic region, *not* the arms.

The lower body should touch the floor from the navel down.

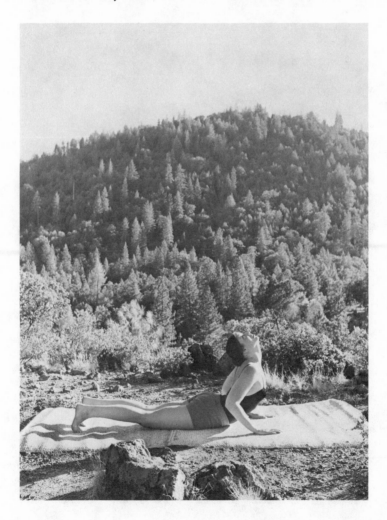

Position 8

A. Exhaling, bring the body back into a pyramid or jackknife pose, as in position 5, shifting the weight so that both the arms and the legs are straight, and the heels are flat on the floor.

B. The head should be face down, directly in line with the arms.

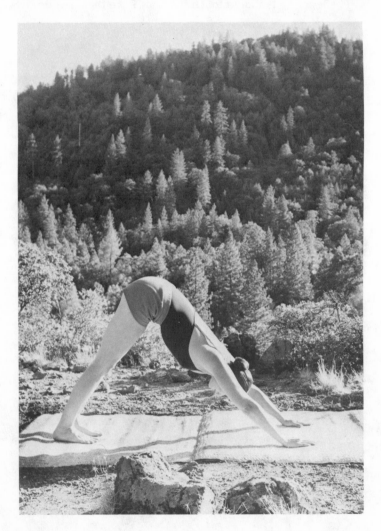

Position 9

A. Inhaling, bring the left leg forward, placing the foot flat between the hands, so that the shin is at a right angle to the floor and the big toe is directly in line with the wrists.

B. At the same time, keeping the palms flat on the floor, raise the head back as far as possible, bending the spine slightly, eyes looking up.

C. The right leg remains stretched behind the body, with the knee touching the floor.

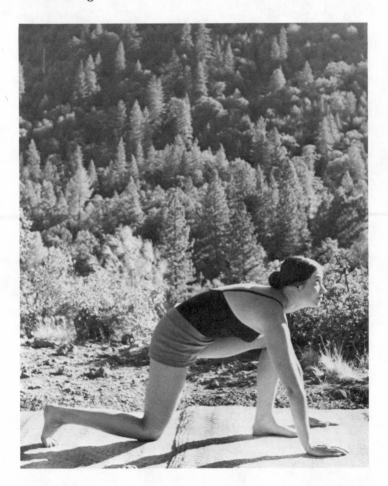

Position 10

A. Exhaling, bring the right leg forward so that the feet are even.

B. The face should touch the knees, the eyes looking toward the stomach and above, and the feet should be kept straight. Palms remain flat on the floor.

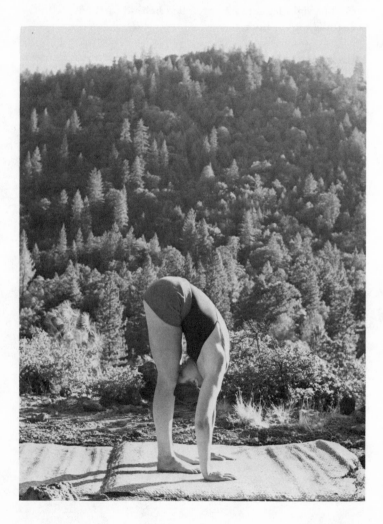

Position 11

A. Inhaling, raise the upper body, lifting the arms outward and upward.

B. Continue the motion until the back is arched and the out-stretched arms are bowed back as far as possible.

C. The head and neck should also be arched, and the elbows kept straight.

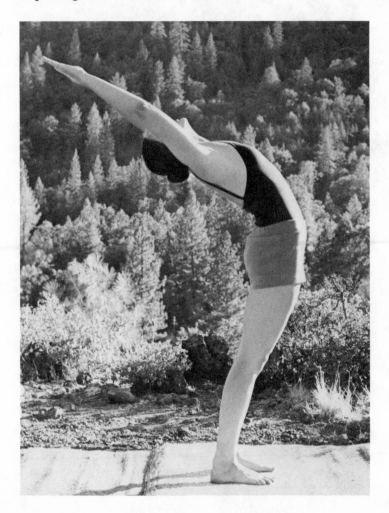

Position 12

A. Exhaling, slowly lower the outstretched arms, resting them at the sides of the body.

B. Relax all the parts of the body in the natural standing posture.

Repeat the cycle of Surya Namaskar a total of 5-25 times, or more if you like.

NOTE: Once the hands and feet are in position, you should not move or shift them to compensate for the difficulty of getting into a pose. And remember the essential keys to posture and movement, as well as the reception-release process of the feeling-breath, and the other disciplines of attention, feeling, and the physical form, which should have been learned from the earlier descriptions.

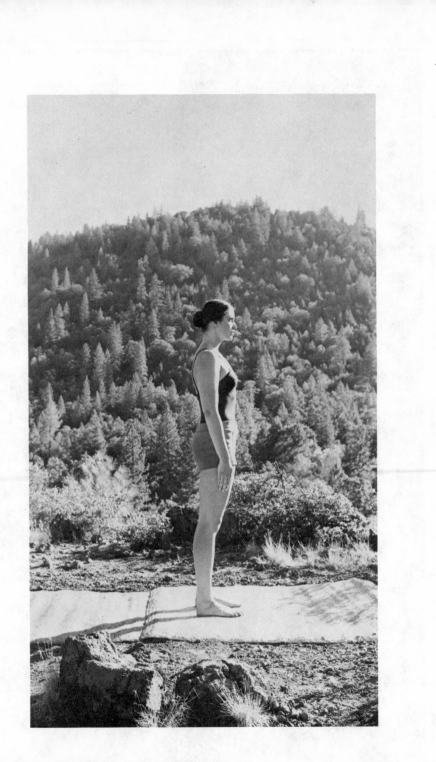

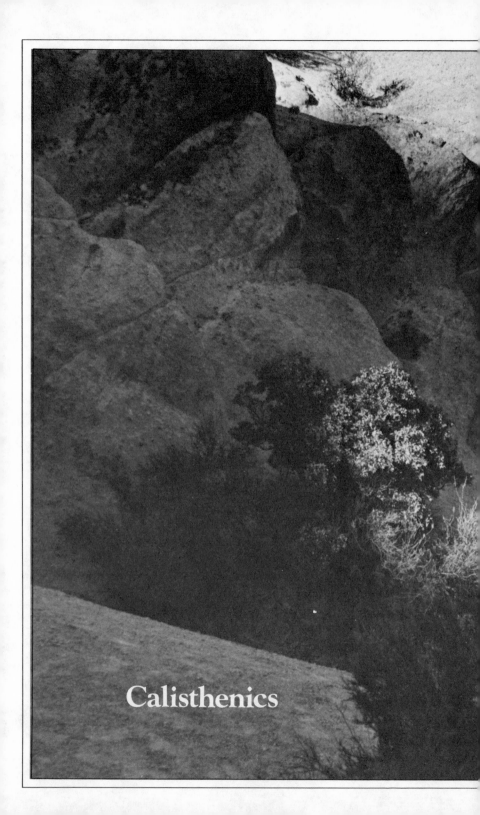

Calisthenics

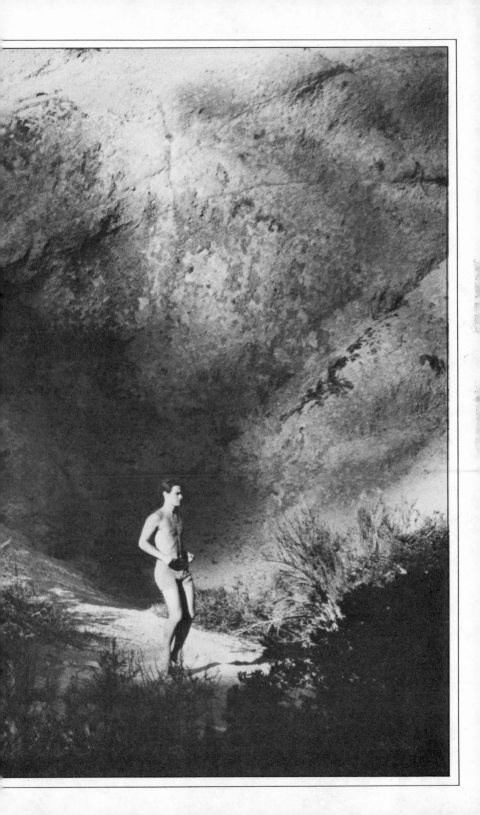

Calisthenics

Points to Remember:

☐ Revitalize the body by conducting the universal life-energy to the vital center, through concentration of feeling-attention in the whole process of exercise, including proper breathing, posture, and the alternating bodily actions of movement and rest, tension and relaxation.

☐ During all conscious exercise, generalized tension is most commonly coupled with intake of breath, and relaxation with exhalation of breath.

☐ You will tend, in performing Calisthenics, to maintain the chronic condition of tension and contraction in the body, and to force the body through the motions of each exercise. But, as in Hatha Yoga, you must *relax* and *feel* the body into these exercises. Even the tensing movements of Calisthenics should be performed with conscious ease and full, relaxed, strong breath.

☐ Do the Calisthenics routine as a continuous, intentional cycle, one exercise after another, to the point of breaking into a light sweat.

☐ Perform each exercise and the whole routine to the point of fullness of energy and feeling, not exhaustion.

☐ Do not mix Calisthenics and Hatha Yoga in the same routine. (However, Surya Namaskar, pages 80-99, should be combined with both Calisthenics and Hatha Yoga.)

☐ Always perform the exercises with the feeling that you are receiving or communing with energy from the living universe, and that you are allowing that energy to permeate the body, mind, and world as you release accumulated psycho-physical patterns of tension and enervation.

☐ Adapt the disciplines of feeling, posture, breathing, "locks," and so forth, as previously described, to the practice of Calisthenics.

☐ The word "Calisthenics" is from the Greek, and signifies an orderly combination or harmony of beauty and strength.

Once you have learned these Calisthenics well, you should feel free to vary or add to them from traditional and contemporary exercise systems. If you modify the order of the exercises, make sure that your sequence balances expansive-stretching movements and contractive-tensing movements of the same parts of the body.

Windmill

A. Stand straight, with the legs spread about two feet apart and toes pointed straight in front of you.

B. Extend arms straight to the sides at shoulder height.

C. Inhale, with great feeling, to the vital center, from the heart, through the nose, via the throat.

D. As you exhale, from the vital center and with the whole body, twist the body from the waist and trunk to the right side until the arms are perpendicular to the axis of the feet and the head is facing behind, the chin pointing along the line of the right arm. The feet should remain stationary. Arms should be extended straight and away from the sides at shoulder height.

E. Inhale, returning the body to its original position.

F. Without breaking the momentum of the body's movement, exhale, twisting the body to the left side in the same manner as above.

The motion of the twist should be fluid and continuous. Repeat the exercise 15 times on each side.

NOTE: Until you are limber and proficient at this exercise, do not twist beyond the point where the arms are directly in line with the axis of the feet. When you are more proficient, you may exercise the body more vigorously by twisting as far as you can to each side, without straining, always keeping the arms straight out from the body. Always twist in a smooth, fluid, and continuous motion.

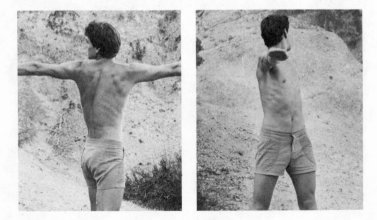

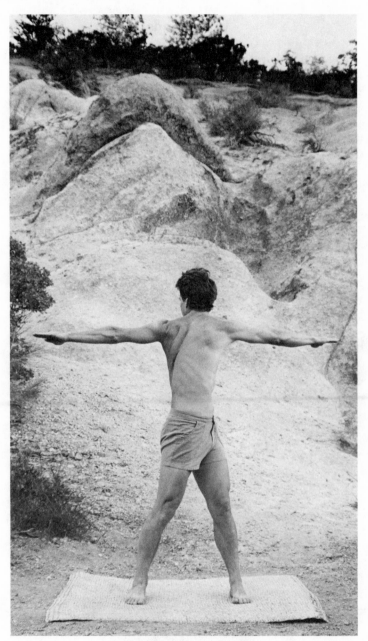

When you are proficient

Waist Bends

A. Stand with feet spread about two feet apart, toes pointing straight ahead, arms extended to the side at shoulder height, eyes looking straight ahead.

B. Inhale, directing breath to the vital center.

C. Exhale, releasing breath from the vital center, bend at the waist, and place the right palm to the ground in front of the left foot.

D. The left arm stays straight out.

E. Inhale as you rise to starting position.

F. Exhale, placing the left palm in front of the right foot, keeping the right arm straight.

G. Inhale, and return to the original position.

Both arms, the head, and the upper trunk should be maintained in their original position throughout this exercise. Bend from the waist. Do not reach to the floor with the hand, but move the whole upper body until the hand naturally touches the floor in the front.

The legs should be kept straight.

Repeat the full exercise (once on each side) 10 times.

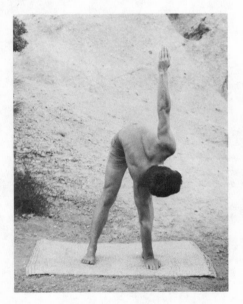

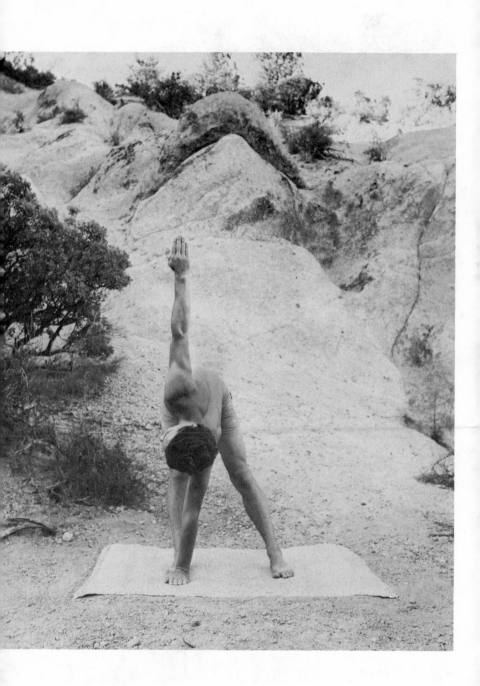

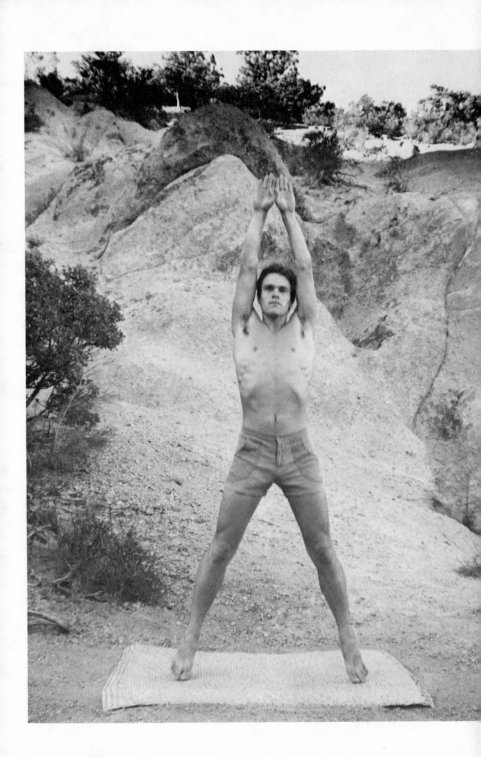

Jumping Jacks

A. Stand erect, feet together and hands to the sides.

B. In one motion, raise the arms straight out to the sides and then above the head so that the hands touch, and at the same time extend the feet about a foot to each side in a jumping motion.

C. Then, again in a single motion, return to the original position, lowering the arms to the sides and bringing the feet back together.

Keep the arms straight throughout this exercise. Perform it rhythmically, with full breathing to and from the vital center.

Repeat 20-25 times.

Walking in Place

A. Stand straight with feet 4-6 inches apart, eyes straight ahead.

B. Twist hips alternately, back and forth—front to back rather than side to side.

The upper part of the body should remain stationary, the knees straight, and the shoulders facing forward.

The arms are bent at the elbows and should move rhythmically, as if you were jogging, but the feet should never leave the floor.

Repeat 20-25 times.

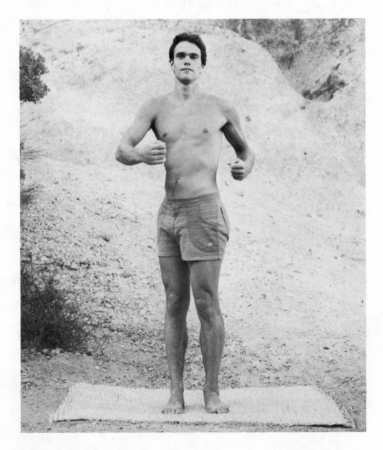

Variations:

1. *Horizontal Rotation*—Stand straight. Relax the arms at the sides or hold them in some other comfortable position, either extended out from the shoulders to one or another degree or relaxed by the sides and bent at the elbows. *Without moving the shoulders or upper body,* rotate the pelvis in a full circle. Do this 10-15 times in one direction, and then 10-15 times in the opposite direction.

2. *Vertical Rotation*—Stand straight, with arms in one of the positions as in Variation 1. Without moving the upper body or the thighs and knees, stretch the pelvis, first forward and up, then back and down, in an "S" or "figure 8" motion. When you are at the "top" of the figure 8, or the peak of the forward and upward motion, the abdominal cavity should naturally become concave, as though pulled in. When extending the pelvis in the outward and downward motion, the abdominal cavity should naturally become convex. The exercise has something of the appearance of "belly dancing," but it is chiefly performed by pelvic motion rather than the abdominal muscles.

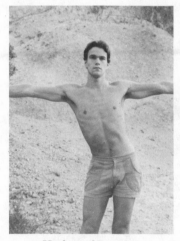

Horizontal Rotation   Vertical Rotation

Knee Bends

A. Stand straight, with the feet spread at about shoulders' width, toes pointing straight ahead.

B. The arms should be extended straight in front of the body at shoulder level. (The hands can also be placed at the waist if you cannot maintain balance with arms extended.)

C. Exhale as you lower the upper body by bending at the knees, squatting as low as possible while keeping the spine straight.

D. The spine should remain erect and the heels of the feet on the ground throughout this exercise.

E. Inhale as you rise to the upright position.

Repeat the exercise 20-25 times, and even increase up to 50 times.

When you are proficient: On several of the Knee Bends, leap off the ground as you rise to the upright position.

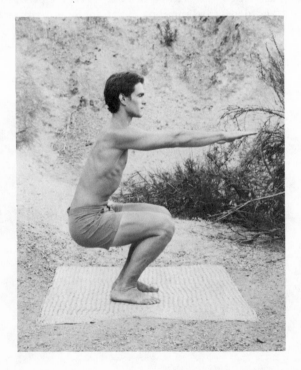

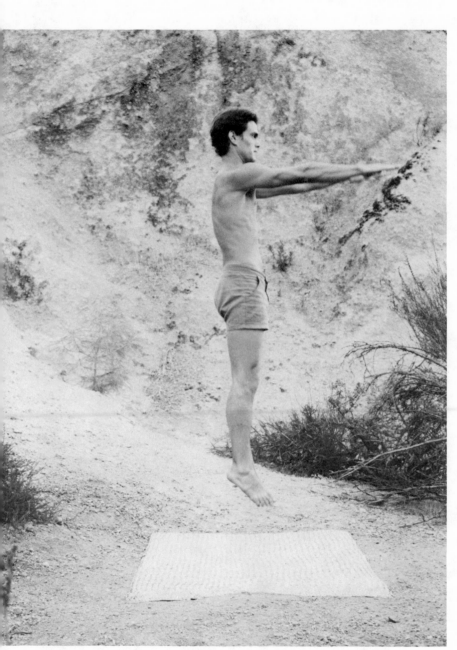

When you are proficient

Running in Place

A. Run in place, making sure that you raise your knees high and lift your heels well off the ground. Arms are bent at the elbows.

B. Running should be rhythmic. Start slowly and gradually build speed, raising the knees to waist level or above at the peak of the exercise.

C. You should run approximately 200-300 steps, increasing speed gradually until your movements are rapid, allowing all body parts to bounce loosely from the spinal axis, then decreasing speed gradually to a stop.

D. Breathe naturally. Breath should be full and directed from the heart to the vital center.

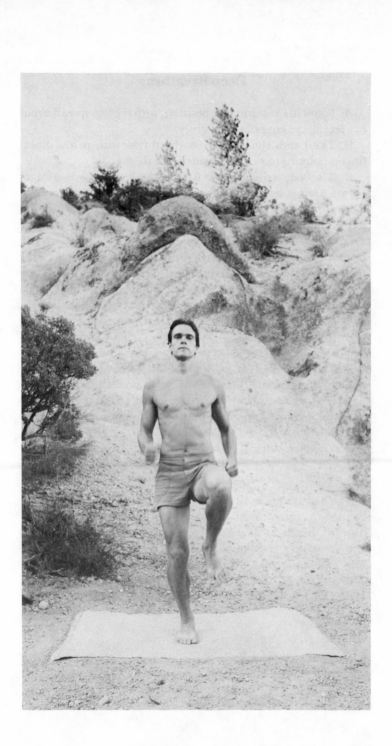

Deep Breathing

A. Stand in a comfortable position, with the legs spread about two feet apart, knees flexed slightly.

B. The hands should rest on the thighs with palms down, fingers pointing toward the inside of the thighs.

C. The body is slightly bent forward at the waist, eyes straight ahead. Do not let the back bow so that the buttocks protrude, but keep the lower back flat and the pelvis pulled forward and slightly tilted up.

D. Inhale, expanding the belly, breathing deeply with full openness of the nostrils, the throat, and the whole trunk of the body, filling the vital center and the whole body.

E. Then exhale quickly, expelling all air from the abdomen and lungs so completely that the whole stomach area becomes a deep cavity. Let the communicated energy pervade the whole body and the world itself. This is one cycle of inhalation and exhalation.

F. The first 5 or 10 cycles should be full and gradually increasing in rapidity. The last few cycles should be slow and full.

G. The tension or upward contraction of the region of the anus-perineum-sex organs is particularly important and useful on exhalation in this exercise.

Practice breathing at least 25-30 cycles.

Variation:

The body position used in the "deep breathing" exercise may be used to exercise the body in motion. While bending slightly forward, hands on thighs or knees, palms down, rotate the hips and spine in a circular motion. Do this several times in one direction, and then an equal number in the opposite direction. The breathing should be in time with the movement, but not in the rapid fashion characteristic of "deep breathing."

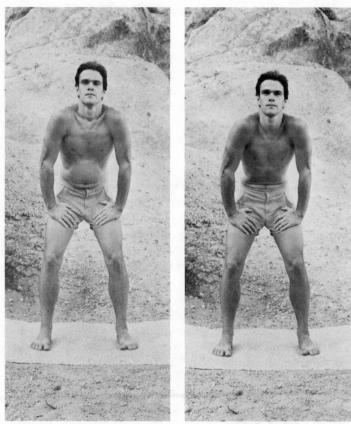

Inhalation   Exhalation

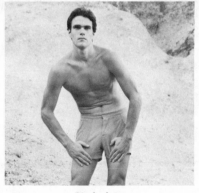

Variation

117

Stomach Roll

A. Stand in a comfortable position, with the feet about two feet apart, resting the hands on the thighs, palms down. The fingers of each hand should be pointing to the inside of the thighs.

B. Lean forward on the hands, applying pressure to both legs.

C. Practice several rounds of deep breathing. (If you can, simply maintain the position you assumed for the Deep Breathing exercise.)

D. Release as much air from the lungs as possible.

E. Relax the stomach muscles, sex organs, and lower body, and then draw them up as if to bring the abdomen back towards the spine and up behind the rib cage, forming a concave stomach and abdomen area.

F. Apply pressure to the right side of the body by pressing the right hand against the right leg, rotating the buttocks to that side slightly.

G. Let the weight of the body shift to the left as the pelvis and buttocks continue the rotating motion.

H. Keep the feet straight and the stomach relaxed. The "roll" will come from rotating the pelvic area, and *not* from applying tension to the stomach area.

I. *The more air you release from the lungs, the easier this exercise.* With exhalation, tilt the pelvis forward and up, and stretch the lower back slightly.

J. Alternate the movement right to left as long as the exhaled breath can be held comfortably.

K. Then repeat, if only a few alternations were achieved.

L. Develop this exercise until you can do 12-15 rounds. (A round includes one movement on each side.)

NOTE: The "Deep Breathing" and "Stomach Roll" exercises are generally considered to be forms of Hatha Yoga, but they work particularly well and combine naturally with routines of Calisthenics.

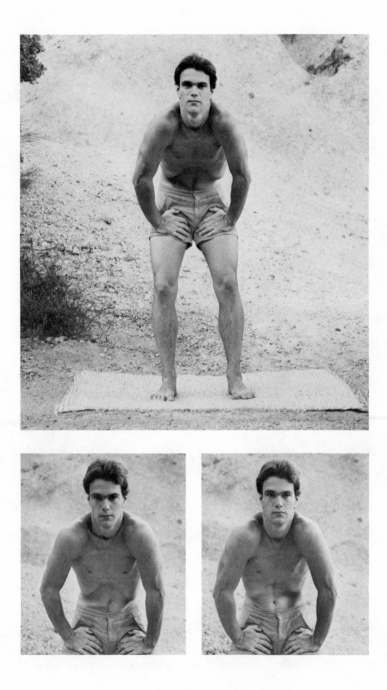

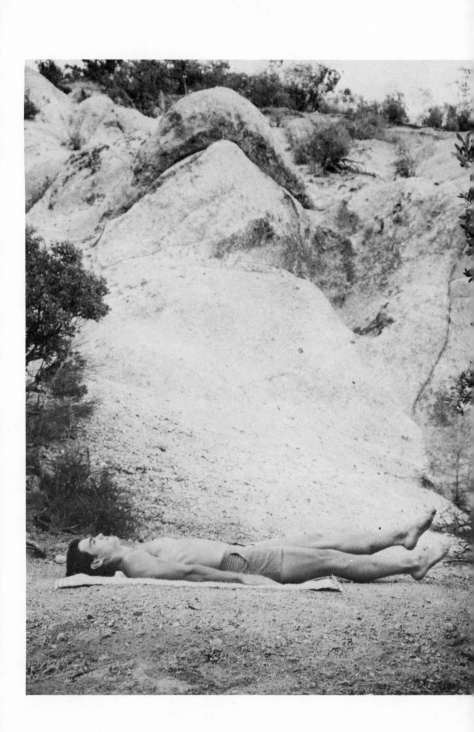

Leg Lifts

A. Lie flat on your back with your arms resting either on the floor straight over the head, or at the sides. (The palms may rest up or down, but if you keep the palms up, you will be less likely to use the hands to assist the legs in the exercise.) The lower back should touch the floor throughout this exercise.

B. Inhale, raising the right leg about one foot off the floor, keeping the knees straight.

C. Bring the right leg down, but do not touch the floor with it, while at the same time exhaling and bringing the left leg up about one foot off the floor.

D. The leg motion is scissor-like and slow, coordinated with the breath. Be sure to keep the legs straight, and do not allow them to touch the floor during this exercise.

Repeat 10-25 times with each leg.

Variation:

A. In the same prone position, bring the right leg up toward the chest, bending it at the knee so that the calf rests on the thigh when the knee is closest to the chest.

B. Then extend that leg forward again while pulling the left leg up to the chest in the same way.

C. Continue in a slow, alternating motion, without letting the feet or legs touch the floor.

Repeat 10-25 times with each leg.

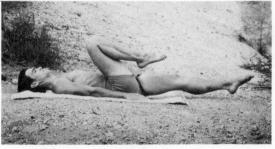

Variation

Sit-Ups

A. Lie flat on the floor with your fingers interlaced behind your head.

B. Keeping your heels and legs flat on the floor, use the abdominal muscles to pull yourself into a sitting position, then continue forward, twisting the trunk to the right to touch the right knee with the left elbow.

C. Then twist the trunk to the left to touch the left knee with the right elbow. (You may reverse the order of these twists.)

D. Using the abdominal muscles to control the motion, return to the prone position.

E. Perform each sit-up as a single, smooth, continuous movement; do not jerk or change speed.

F. The legs should always lie straight ahead, flat on the floor.

G. Inhale just before you begin, exhale as you sit up, and inhale again as you lie down.

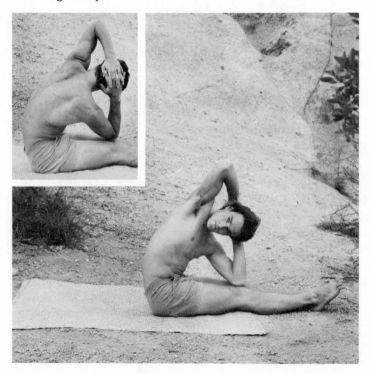

Variations:

1. A more difficult version of this exercise can be done with the arms extended straight behind the head in the prone position.

When moving forward from the sitting position, press the face between the knees and let the hands drop forward at the sides of the feet.

Begin by doing only a few sit-ups, but gradually increase the repetitions to 10 or 15.

It is generally recommended that you practice with the hands locked behind the head, touching the elbows to the opposite knees, until you are limber enough for this version.

Other variations of this exercise include:

2. Use a slant board with the feet elevated (not shown).

3. Keep the knees bent with the feet flat on the floor and touch the elbows to the knees alternately.

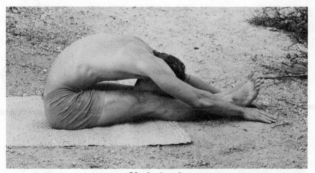

Variation 1

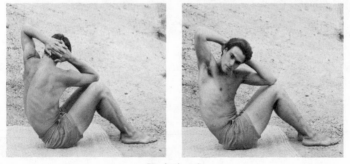

Variation 3

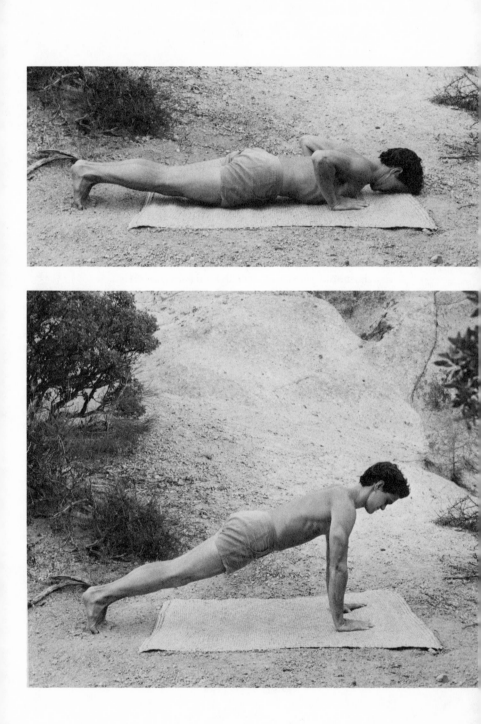

Push-Ups

A. Lie on the stomach with the hands resting palms down directly under the shoulders, fingers straight and the toes gripping the floor.

B. To begin, straighten the arms, raising the body off the floor as you inhale. The entire body should be completely straight, making a single angle with the floor, with the head, back, buttocks, thighs, and calves in a single straight line.

C. When the arms are fully extended, the elbows should be locked into place.

D. Then exhale, lowering the body so that the chest and forehead touch the floor lightly.

Be sure *not* to let the stomach or knees touch the floor during this exercise. Push-ups should number 15-20 when you are proficient.

Push-ups for women: Women may elect to modify this exercise by resting the lower body on the knees, rather than the toes, holding the feet together and above the floor, and then performing the exercise as described above.

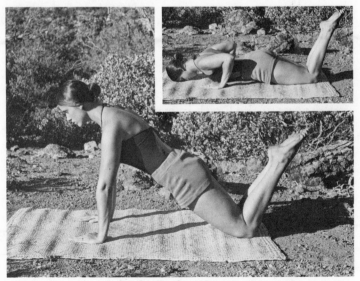

Push-Ups for Women

Twirling and Jet Lag: A Way to Equalize the Effects of the Earth's Rotation and of Fast Transportation, by Bubba Free John

Twirling is a natural exercise in which the physical (elemental) body and its etheric energy field are realigned and reintegrated, thereby equalizing or refreshing the living being. This is done in two ways: (1) Through the generation of feeling-attention in the exercise, the etheric is made to fully pervade the elemental, and (2) through the action or movement of twirling, the elemental and the etheric are made into a single vortex, whereby they become equalized or integrated in a mutual harmony, a common "speed."

The two sides of the body represent two tendencies (expansive and passive) in play, wherein one or the other may be dominant in any moment. Just so, the whole theatre of manifest existence in which we appear bodily is a like play of opposites, and we experience the effects of this play in different ways from moment to moment.

Earth itself is a perpetual twirling machine. The human body standing on Earth is aligned to the twirling process of the Earth in every moment. It is appropriate, therefore, for us to be consciously responsible for the effects of this association and for a right or harmonious integration with the whole process in which it all appears.

Earth and the human body each represent the same machine of motion and polarization. Earth has a north pole and a south pole. These correspond to the head and the feet of every human individual. At the equator of the Earth we refer to the east and the west directions. These correspond to the left hand

and the right hand of every human individual. If you were to imagine yourself to be a weather vane, you would see how the head, the feet, and the two arms correspond to the four directions and duplicate the polarities of Earth itself.

The sun appears to move from east to west, because the Earth is "twirling" or rotating from west to east. Since we all appear and stand on the Earth and, whether consciously or unconsciously, constantly duplicate its condition as well as experience and reflect the effects of its motion and polarization, it is as if we ourselves are constantly twirling west to east, or right over left.

The motion of the physical or elemental Earth itself is tending toward its own center. It is the motion that creates pressure toward the center, that moves from a diffused condition toward a point or a defined condition. Every human individual is likewise so disposed. Earth and the human individual are a synchronous or simultaneous machine. Thus, the natural effect the Earth's twirling has on man is to reinforce his orientation toward self and subjectivity, defined or limited by his elemental or gross bodily form. The right side (the "west") of the human body is associated with the expansive and outward tendency, and the left side (the "east") with the passive or inward tendency. Thus, if in effect we are always twirling in circles, right toward left, the expansive tendency, toward diffusion, is constantly yielding toward the contracting tendency, toward bodily definition. For this reason, intense participation in personal, bodily or "worldly" concerns tends to make us feel "up tight." We are always tending to become defined, limited, and self-possessed.

The conscious exercise of twirling is a way to participate in the polarizations and motions of the Earth-born body, so that the effects of the Earth's process and our own random activity may be counter-balanced or equalized in a simple manner.

The motion of the Earth and the sympathies of man are tending toward Earthly confinement, or the definition of our existence by the elemental body. The etheric or energy dimension of Earth and our own body is, in contrast, tending more toward an expanded or diffused condition. The integration of the two tendencies yields a harmony, a pleasurable equalization, which is effectively at rest.

We may twirl as an expression of this process of equalization. Since we are in effect always twirling right toward left, we may counter this by twirling left toward right. Then the passive-contractive yields into the active-expansive disposition, to the point of balance or equalization.

Particularly when you feel "up tight" (contracted), twirl left to right, with a fully expansive and radiant feeling, as in conscious exhalation. When you feel more enervated or "washed out," twirl right to left, with a feeling of being infilled, collected, centered, and intensified, as in conscious inhalation.

Twirling is, secondarily, also an excellent remedy for "jet lag." If you have flown in an eastward direction, twirl westward (left over right). If you have flown westward, twirl eastward (right over left). Do this several times, and also rest awhile, after flying in an airplane, or even traveling by automobile or some other faster-than-human transportation. Fast travel sets up a motion in our energy-feeling system that takes a little time to return to human speed. Therefore, rest at least briefly in the "Dead Pose" after travel, and twirl several times every hour or so after traveling in a conveyance.

Daily life in cities and in occupations or environments that involve rapid movement or rapid communication requires us consciously to counter the effects with relaxation repose. As an adjunct to the activities whereby we equalize the tendencies of our ordinary functional life, twirling may become an important form of conscious exercise.

Twirl with great feeling and abandon, while yet controlling the movement and avoiding dizzy collapse. Twirl in a small space. That is, keep the feet on the same spot rather than skate around the room. Rest afterwards, and repeat again.

Twirling right over left generally tends to energize us or concentrate energy. Twirling left over right generally tends to relax us or expand our energy.

All space, the moon and stars, the clouds and sky, the sun itself and what is beyond are objects of our expansive interest, whereby we counter the effects of our busy Earth-consciousness and self-consciousness. Therefore, always be alive to what you do not yet or ever can possess and know. Wonder rests the vital being and cools the brain. When you are free to know nothing and be nothing, then you may hear what is Truth, and so become a devotee of the Unknown through eternal and always present Ignorance.

Twirling

A. Stand erect, facing straight ahead, with arms extended straight out to the sides (parallel to the front of the body) at shoulder level.

B. Spin or twirl the body in a clockwise direction (left toward right), with great feeling.

C. Generally, keep the eyes open and turned straight ahead as you twirl. (As a variation, you may also try twirling with eyes closed.)

D. The head, arms, and upper body should be held erect in the original position throughout this exercise.

E. The breathing should be full, to and from the vital center.

F. The feet should essentially remain in the same area.

G. You can twirl as many times as you like, or you can twirl 10-12 times, stop, and then begin another cycle.

H. Avoid collapsing and falling down, if possible. Thus, remain standing at the completion of each cycle, looking straight ahead in one direction, and allow the composure of the body to return.

I. *After* the visual and other bodily effects of spinning and dizziness have ended, lie down and begin the Dead Pose.

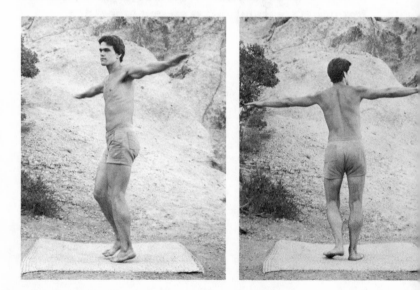

Twirling can be done at the end of both the morning Calisthenics routine and the Hatha Yoga routine, and randomly at any other time throughout the day. If you maintain proper breathing and full feeling-attention to the whole process, you will not feel overly-profound dizziness after the first few times you practice this exercise.

It is generally recommended that you twirl in a clockwise direction (left toward right), to counter the contractive, defining, limiting tendency that is constantly created and reinforced by the general trend of experience. But any time you are feeling enervated or uncollected, you may try twirling in the opposite direction, counter-clockwise (right toward left). Some people, especially those who are generally not very well "grounded," or who are chronically tending toward enervation, may prefer twirling in this counter-clockwise direction regularly. Anyone may prefer to do so simply because it feels better; experiment for yourself. And you may find it useful after traveling via fast mechanical transportation (moving a long distance in a short time) to twirl and rest—left over right if you have traveled eastward or feel "up tight," and right over left if you have traveled westward or feel tired out.

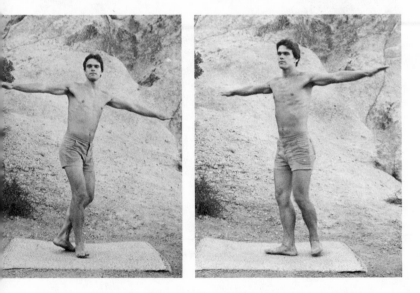

Dead Pose

A. Lie on your back with the legs extended and spread comfortably apart, and with the arms extended to either side of the body at a comfortable distance.

B. Close the circuits of the hands by touching each thumb and forefinger.

C. Completely, and with deep feeling, relax each part of the body in ascending order, beginning with the toes and including all the muscles, the ligaments, each internal organ, the stomach, lungs, heart, the entire surface of the skin, even the teeth, eyes, forehead, hair, and brain.

D. Maintain normal breathing (filling on inhalation, permeating on exhalation), remaining in the pose for up to 3-4 minutes or longer, or until the breath is even and you feel relaxed and energized.

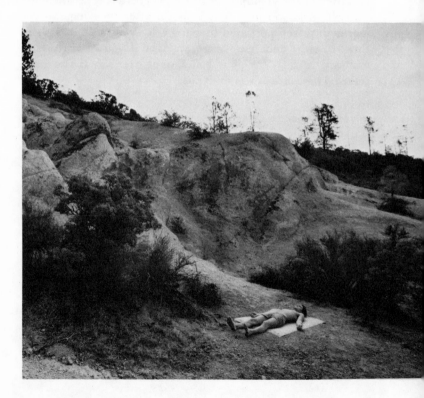

Variations:

1. Tense the whole body, even clenching the fists, while inhaling, then exhale and completely and feelingly relax the body.

Do this 2 or 3 times at the beginning of the pose, and then continue as indicated above.

2. Another variation of the Dead Pose is to cross one of the ankles over the other, and otherwise to follow the original instructions. (Generally, crossing the left ankle over the right creates a "relaxation circuit" of energy for most people. However, some prefer the reverse, that is, crossing the right ankle over the left. Experiment to determine which is more relaxing for you.)

3. A third variation of the Dead Pose is the "Vacation Pose." Clasp the hands behind the head, with arms resting on the floor, cross the legs at the ankles, and proceed with the exercise as indicated above. (This variation is helpful in breaking up tension in the neck and shoulder region.)

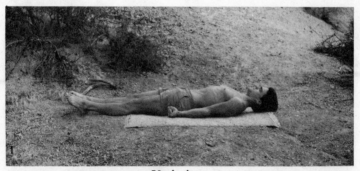

Variations

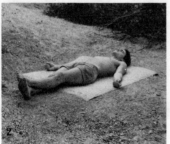
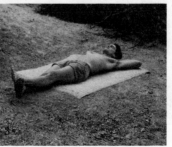

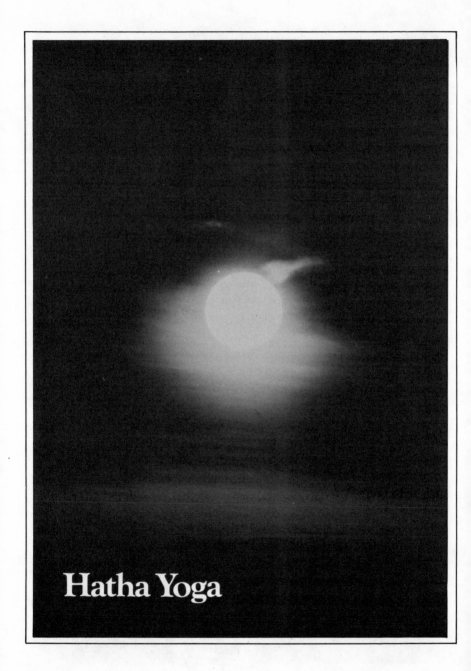

Hatha Yoga

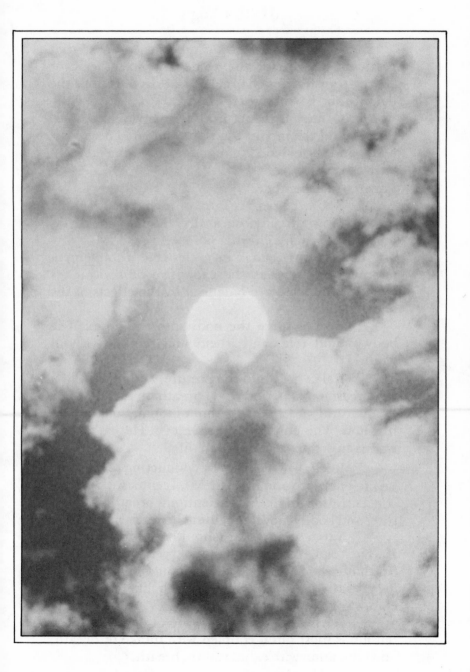

Hatha Yoga

Hatha Yoga is a system of poses or "asanas" that particularly exercise the spine and its etheric or energy-transferring channels. It works to restore the balance and harmony of the body.

"Hatha" means the natural harmony of opposites, the sun and the moon, the right and left sides of the body, and the exhaled (expansive) and inhaled (centering) breaths.

Points to Remember:

☐ Know the perfect form of each pose or asana.

☐ Move directly, naturally, fluidly, and rhythmically into each following pose.

☐ Perform asanas in cycles that complement one another, so that the expansive or contractive effects of any pose are balanced by the effects of the one that follows.

☐ Do not force the body into the poses. The body should relax into them and remain without strain.

☐ Relax fully into the posture, and remain in it for a reasonable period while breathing the life-force in a natural and *equal* rhythm of inhalation and exhalation. This equality is the secret of Hatha Yoga as well as an ordinary harmonious life.

☐ Revitalize the body by conducting the universal life-energy to and from the vital center with proper concentration of feeling-attention, breathing, posture, and bodily movement in each exercise.

☐ Surya Namaskar should be done before Hatha Yoga, to limber and oxygenate the body. (In that case, Surya Namaskar should be performed in a relatively easy manner, much like a series of Hatha Yoga exercises.)

☐ During all conscious exercise, generalized tension is most often coupled with intake of breath, and relaxation with exhalation of breath.

☐ Do not mix Calisthenics and Hatha Yoga in the same routine.

☐ Always hold poses or asanas to the degree of pleasure or need. The body itself will let you know when to release the pose.

☐ And always perform the exercise with the feeling that you are receiving harmonizing energy and releasing all negative and contracted conditions of body, emotion, and mind.

☐ It is generally recommended that women do not practice the inverted poses (Headstand, The Plow, etc.) during the menstrual period, as these poses may tend to interrupt the natural flow in the body and create a disharmony.

☐ After you become proficient, you may wish to vary the sequence of poses outlined below. Some people, for instance, prefer to practice the Headstand before, rather than after, the forward-stretching poses and the Plow-Shoulder Stand-Bridge sequence (see pages 154-160) to give the neck and spine a full stretch.

In the beginning, poses should generally be done in the order given here, since the order has been created to balance complementary poses and provide a rhythmic progression. Once you have learned them well, you should feel free to vary their order and number, and you may also add to them from the traditional sources in ways that feel appropriate to you. The primary rule in doing so is always to remember to balance contractive poses with expansive poses (and vice versa), in a natural rhythm or sequence that stretches the same parts of the body in opposite ways.

A number of the poses in the basic Hatha Yoga routine depend upon your capacity to assume one or more of the sitting poses traditionally used for meditation. Instructions for the sitting poses are given on pages 175-189.

Trunk Roll

A. Stand straight.

B. Raise the arms straight up over the head, fingers extended.

C. Begin to rotate the outstretched arms, hands, and upper body in a counter-clockwise circular motion above the head, tracing a circle 2-3 feet in diameter. It is important that the arms and hands remain outstretched straight above the head during the entire exercise.

D. The hips and torso should rotate in a circular motion in

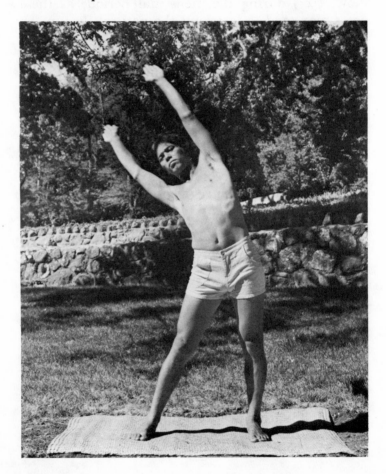

rhythmic coordination with the outstretched arms. The knees should be kept straight.

E. Inhale as you arch the back in rotating motion, and exhale as you bend forward.

Repeat 10 times or more, then rotate in the opposite direction an equal number of times.

Variation (without rotation):

A. Stand in a comfortable position with the feet 8-10 inches apart.

B. Stretch the arms straight above the head, inhaling as you do so.

C. Exhale, stretching both arms laterally to the right side of the body as far as possible.

D. Inhale, returning to the starting position, and repeat on the opposite side.

Remain in each side stretch 10-15 seconds or more.

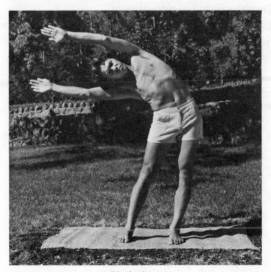

Variation

Tree Pose

A. Stand in a comfortable position, facing forward, toes pointed straight ahead.

B. Bend the right leg, place the right heel on the left thigh close to the groin, and let the top of the foot rest on the thigh, keeping the left leg straight.

C. Turn the right knee downward.

D. Lift both arms above the head, keeping the elbows straight and bringing the palms together.

E. Once in this pose, relax fully. The body should remain erect.

Remain in this pose for 1-2 minutes or longer.

Repeat the pose using the opposite leg.

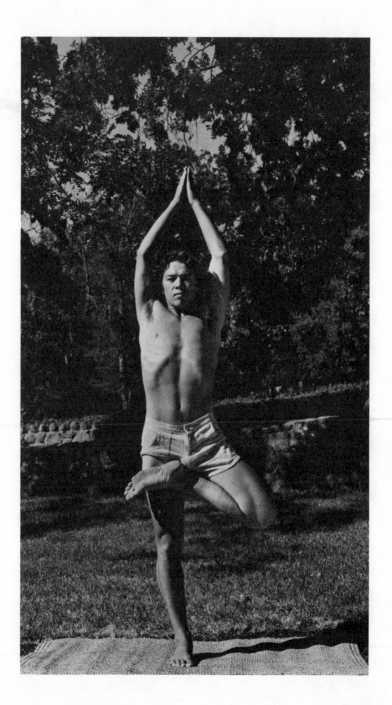

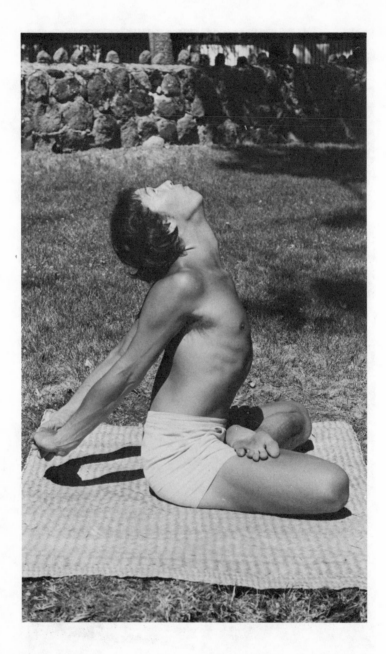

Variation in Lotus Pose or Half-Lotus Pose

A. Sit in the Lotus or Half-Lotus Pose. (See pages 177-181 for instructions on these sitting poses.)

B. Extend the arms behind you, locking the fingers together with the palms up.

C. With your locked hands, stretch the arms down toward the floor as if to pull the head back.

D. Inhale.

E. Lift the chin and let the head be pulled back as far as possible, eyes looking above.

F. Hold the breath as you maintain this pose for 10-15 seconds.

G. Exhale slowly and return to the normal sitting pose.

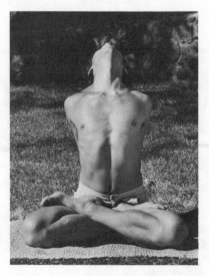

Downward Neck Pull

A. Sit in the Lotus Pose or the Half-Lotus Pose, with the spine straight.

B. Place the palm of either hand on the crown of the head.

C. Exhaling through the nose, slowly pull the head down so that the chin rests snugly into the jugular notch at the top of the chest and the force of the stretch can be felt all the way down the spine.

D. Keep the spine straight.

E. Remain in this pose for 15 seconds or more, breathing normally.

F. Raise the head slowly to an upright position.

Variation:

This pose also works very well if done in a squatting position.

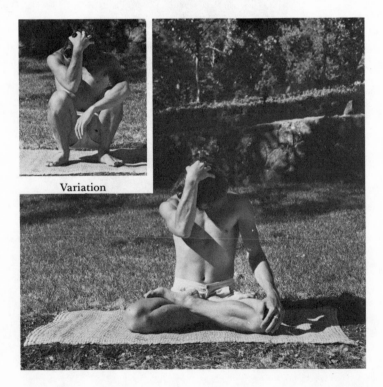

Variation

Neck Roll

A. Sit in the Lotus Pose or the Half-Lotus Pose, with the hands in the lap and the eyes closed.

B. Relax the neck muscles and allow the head to fall forward as if it were a dead weight.

C. Slowly rotate the head in a full circular motion. Begin slowly and increase the speed.

D. Rotate the head as many as 10 times or more, decreasing the speed gradually.

E. Balance this exercise by rotating the head in the opposite direction in the same manner.

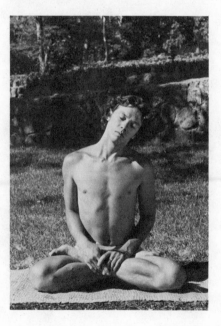

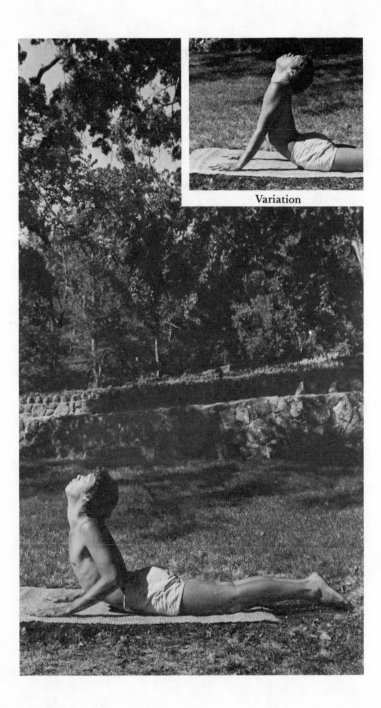

Variation

The Cobra

A. Lie on the stomach, placing the palms on the floor at the sides of the body, even with the shoulders. Relax the body.

B. Inhale as you slowly roll the head upward, and raise the upper portion of the body with the arms, so that the back is arched in such a way that the pelvic bones remain on the floor and the head is pulled back as far as possible.

C. Do not straighten the arms fully, but hold them as straight as you can without lifting the upper abdomen off the floor.

D. Legs should be straight and relaxed.

E. Hold the breath and remain in the pose for 8-10 seconds, or longer if you like.

F. Exhale and slowly return to the original position.

Variation:

A. Perform the exercise as above, but arch the whole spine backward, so that the whole upper abdomen to the pubic bone is lifted off the floor.

B. Arms should be as straight as possible.

C. When you are proficient at this variation, you should be able to lock the arms at the elbows while holding the pose.

The Bow

A. Lie on the stomach, bending both legs at the knee.

B. Grasp the left ankle with the left hand and the right ankle with the right hand.

C. As you inhale, raise the head, torso, and legs so that the back is arched. Pull the legs at the ankles so that the thighs are raised off the ground. The weight of the body should be on the abdominal-pelvic area, and head and neck should be arched as far backward as possible.

D. Retain the breath while in this pose.

E. Hold the pose for 10-15 seconds or more.

F. Exhale, and lower the body to the floor.

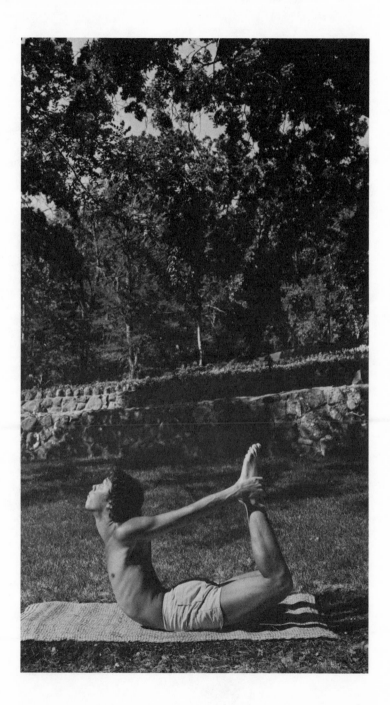

The Locust

A. Lie on the stomach, resting the chin on the floor. Arms should be at your sides, palms up.

B. Clench both hands into fists, inhale, and stiffen the whole body, raising both legs straight off the floor, keeping the knees straight.

C. Keeping the chin on the floor, arch the back to allow the legs and upper thighs to go as high off the floor as possible.

D. Remain in this pose for 7-8 seconds or more.

E. Slowly exhale and lower the legs to the floor.

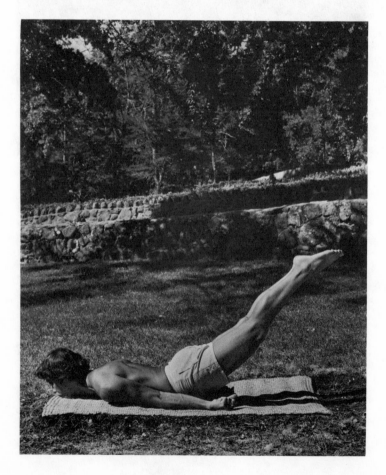

Forward Stretching Pose

A. Sit in an upright position with the legs extended, knees together, and the back straight.

B. Inhale, extending the arms straight above the head.

C. Exhale while bending forward from the waist and clasping the toes. (A comfortable way to do this pose is to grasp the big toes with the thumb and forefinger of each hand.) The breath should be fully expelled.

D. Keeping the knees flat to the ground, continue bending forward until the nose or the whole face touches the knees. (If you cannot touch the knees with any part of your face, then hold the nose as close to that position as possible without strain.)

Remain in the pose for 10-15 seconds or longer.

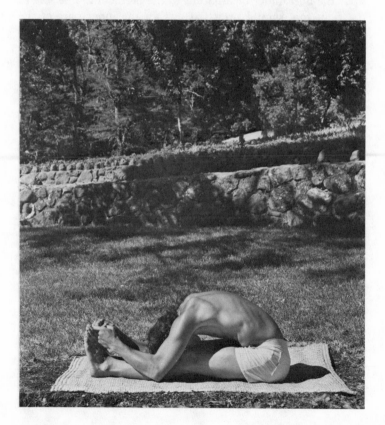

Head to Knees Pose

A. Sit in an upright position with the legs together and extended straight ahead, thighs and calves flat on the floor, and the back straight, as at the beginning of the Forward Stretching Pose.

B. Bend the right leg at the knee, grasp the right foot, and press the heel under or adjacent to the perineum. The sole of the right foot should press flat against the inner part of the left thigh.

C. The whole right leg, including the knee, should now be flat on the floor. It should remain in that position throughout the exercise.

D. Rest the arms at the sides and relax briefly in the fully upright position, with the back straight.

E. Inhale, extending the arms straight above the head, as in the Forward Stretching Pose.

F. Exhale, bending forward from the waist and clasping the left big toe with the fingers of both hands.

G. Keeping the left leg straight and flat on the floor, continue bending forward until the nose touches the left knee. (If you cannot touch the knee with your nose, then hold the nose as close to that position as possible without strain.)

H. Hold the pose for 10-15 seconds or longer.

I. Return to the original position and repeat, this time with the left leg bent and its heel under or adjacent to the perineum.

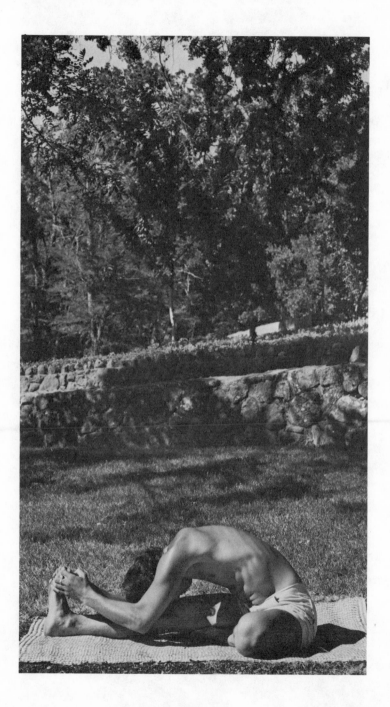

The Plow

Move into this pose directly from the Head to Knees Pose.

A. Recline the upper body backward to the floor and bring the legs up and over the head.

B. Lower the feet to the floor behind the head until the toes are able to grip the floor.

C. The legs should be kept straight throughout the exercise, and the chin should be tucked into the jugular notch.

D. The arms should rest on the floor straight out behind the head.

Remain in this pose for 2-3 minutes or longer.

Variation:

A. Still in the Plow, bend the knees so they touch the ground beside the ears.

B. Fold the arms around the legs, or rest them to the sides.

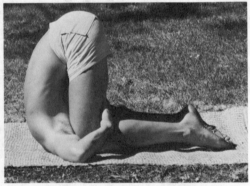

Variation

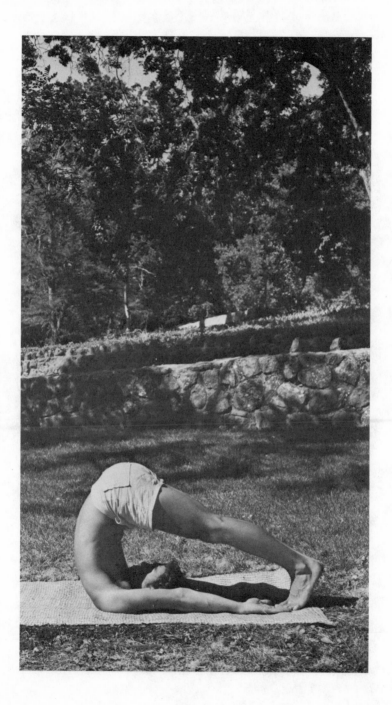

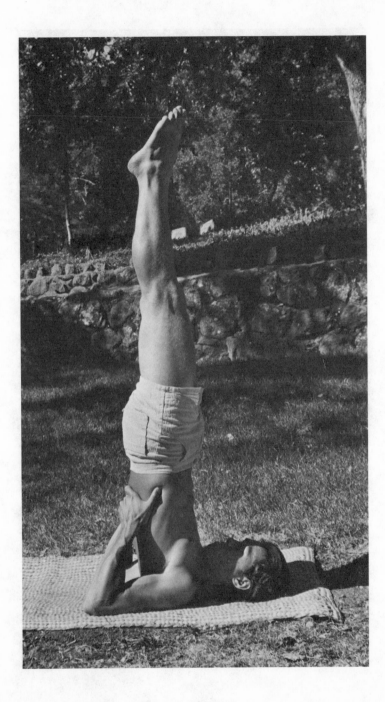

Shoulder Stand

A. Lie on the back with the legs together and arms at the sides.

B. Raise both feet off the floor, keeping the legs straight and together.

C. Continue to lift the feet over the head and raise the back off the floor, supporting it with the hands and elbows.

D. The body should be as straight as possible, resting vertically on the shoulders, and the weight should be on the back of the neck and the back part of the head, with the chin pressing into the jugular notch of the chest.

E. Relax in this pose for one minute or longer.

F. Return to the prone position by simply reversing the procedure you followed in moving into the posture.

Variation (without hands):

Perform the Shoulder Stand as instructed above.

A. Once the body is in the vertical position, remove the hands from the waist and let the arms rest at the sides, without strained support of any of the body's weight.

B. When returning to the prone position, you may use the hands and arms for support or not, according to your preference and the body's strength.

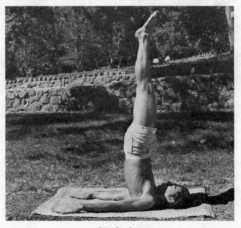

Variation

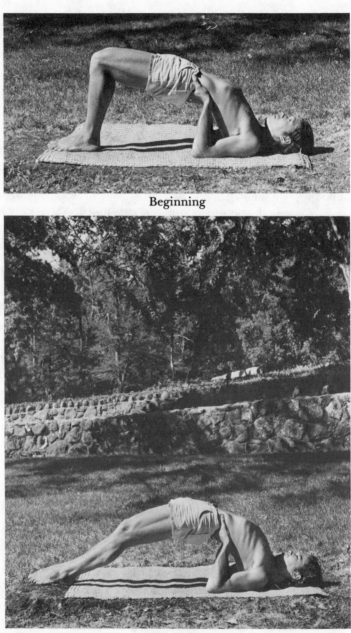

Beginning

Advanced

The Bridge

A. Lie on your back.

B. With the feet flat on the floor, raise the knees, and, keeping them together, lift your hips off the floor so that the back is arched as high as possible.

C. Bring the feet close to the hips, while still keeping the shoulders flat on the floor.

D. Supporting your back with your hands at your waist gives a better arch to the spine.

As your back becomes stronger you can begin to move the feet away from the body. In the advanced Bridge Pose the knees are straight and the feet and legs together, so that the body is a smooth arch from the shoulders to the feet.

In the beginning you may find it more comfortable to keep the feet closer to the body and rest the arms against the floor.

Deep, full breathing in this pose helps clear the lungs.

Hold the pose for 15-30 seconds.

Advanced Method of Assuming the Bridge Pose

When the body is strong, the Bridge can be done from the Shoulder Stand. A succession of Plow, Shoulder Stand and Bridge gives a pleasurable stretch in both directions to the entire spine.

A. While in the Shoulder Stand, support the back with the hands at the waist.

B. Keeping the legs as straight as possible, slowly lower your feet to the floor so that the back is arched over the hands.

C. Keep the elbows as close together as possible for a greater stretch.

When you are more proficient, extend the feet and press the hands upwards, arching the back.

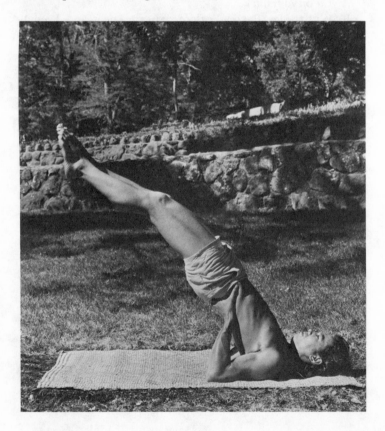

The Fish

A. Sit in the Lotus.

B. Arch the back and, supporting the body with hands and forearms, lower the body backward slowly to the floor, resting the top of the head on the floor.

C. Relax, letting the arms rest at the sides of the body and placing the hands on the feet.

D. The weight of the body should be on the top of the head and on the buttocks, *not* on the elbows.

Remain relaxed in the pose for one minute or more.

Deep, full breathing in this pose helps to clear the lungs.

It is also good to relax briefly in the Dead Pose (page 132) after this stage in the routine before going on to the other poses.

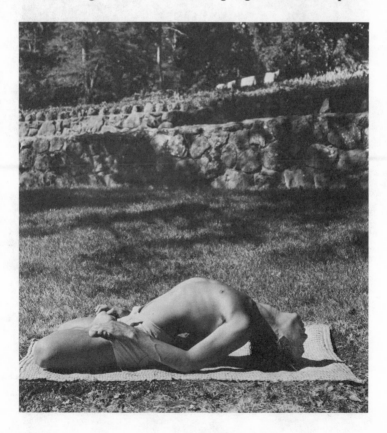

The Peacock

A. Assume a kneeling position.

B. Place the arms together in front of you, with the palms on the floor and the fingers facing toward the toes.

C. Lower the stomach into the elbows, balancing on the forearms and hands.

D. Inhale, and raise the legs parallel to the floor. Keep the legs straight.

Remain in the pose for 10-15 seconds or longer.

This pose may be too difficult for most women.

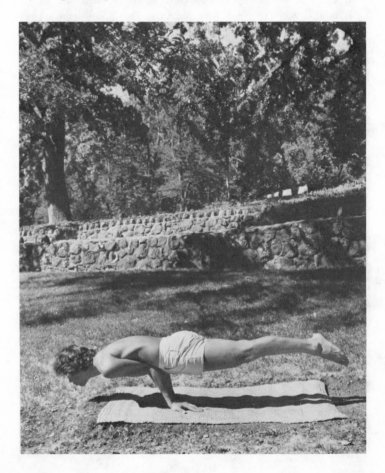

The Wheel

A. Assume a kneeling position, with the feet outstretched and the ankles and tops of the feet flat on the floor.

B. Reach back with each hand and grasp the corresponding ankle.

C. Inhale and arch the body from the waist, bending backward as far as possible.

D. Keep the arms straight throughout this pose, and remain in it for 15-30 seconds or longer.

E. With the exhalation, come back to the upright position.

Variation:

Assume a kneeling position, but place the feet at right angles to the floor, with the toes flat on the floor. Then perform the exercise as instructed above.

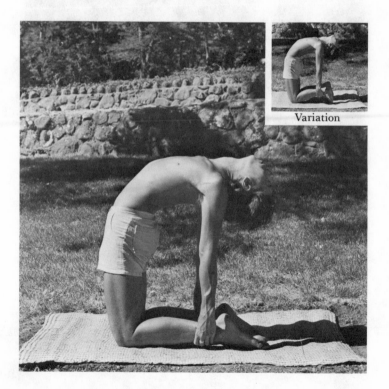

Variation

163

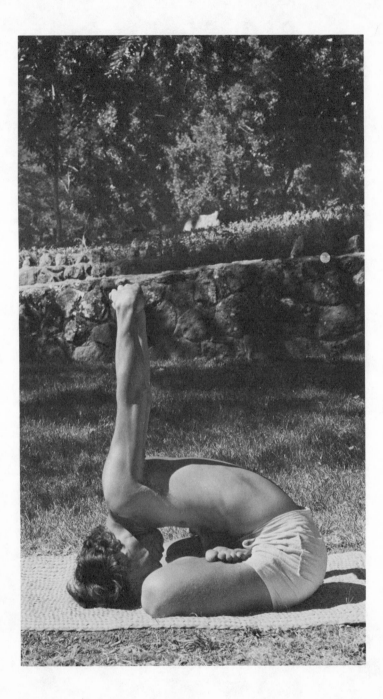

The Forward Bending Lotus

A. Sit in the Lotus or the Half-Lotus.

B. Clasp the hands behind you on the floor.

C. Exhaling fully, bend forward at the waist, allowing the top of the head to touch the floor and causing the chin to press into the jugular notch.

D. At the same time, keeping the hands clasped, extend the arms straight up as far as possible. The movements of the trunk, head, and arms (C and D) should be coordinated as a single motion.

E. Remain in this pose for 10-15 seconds or longer without inhaling.

F. Then inhale as you return to the starting position.

Variation:

Perform the exercise as stated here, but bow at the waist from a standing position. When the pose is fully assumed:

A. The nose or the whole face should touch the knees, and

B. The eyes should look up toward the navel.

This version of the Forward Bending Lotus gives a greater stretch to the lower back and also the shoulders and arms.

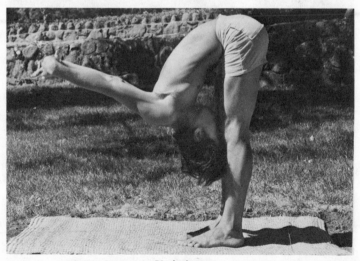

Variation

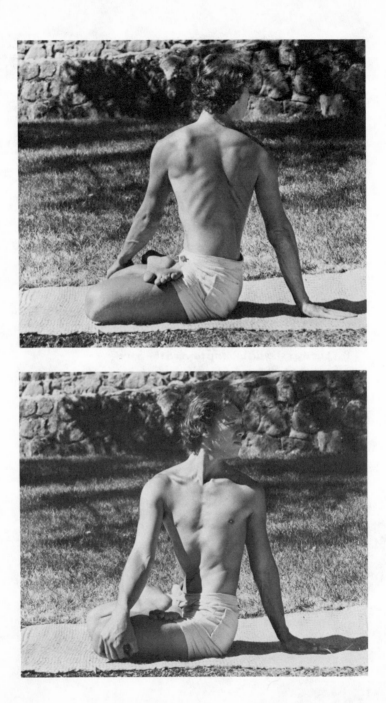

Spinal Twist

A. Sit in the Lotus or the Half-Lotus.

B. The left hand should hold the right knee, and the right hand should be flat on the floor directly behind you, approximately a foot away from the spine.

C. Using the hand on the knee as a fulcrum, twist the upper body and neck as far to the right as possible, exhaling as you do so, keeping the chest and head erect, and hold the pose briefly.

D. Do the same on the left side. Once on each side is usually sufficient. You may experience an enjoyable (and harmless) cracking of the spine.

The Lion Pose

Phase 1:

A. Assume a kneeling position, resting the buttocks on the heels, with the hands resting on the knees.

B. As you exhale fully, stretch the tongue out and down as far as possible, while at the same time rolling the eyes up into the head as far as you can.

C. Tense the body and stretch the fingers outward as the palms rest on the knees.

Remain in this pose 10-15 seconds or longer.

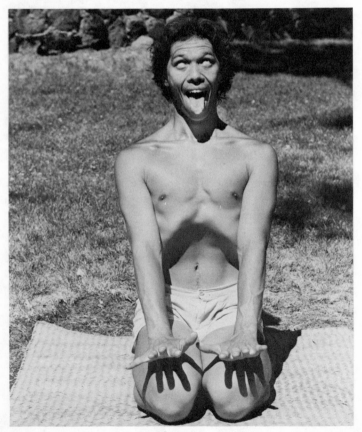

Phase 1

Phase 2:

Balance the first form of the Lion Pose by exhaling and stretching the tongue out and up, touching the nose if possible. This time, the eyes should be turned downward.

Do the complementary pose for a period of time equal to that of the original Lion Pose.

Variation:

In either or both of the two Phases of the Lion Pose, the eyes may be rotated, first in one direction and then the other, rather than simply held in an upward or downward direction.

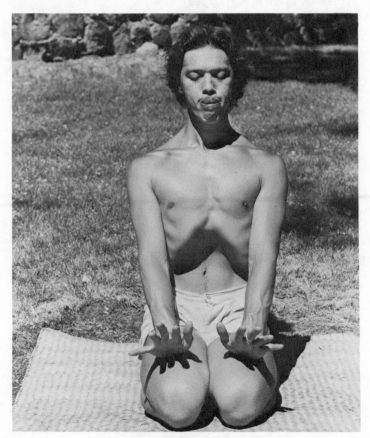

Phase 2

Headstand

A. Assume a kneeling position.

B. Bend over and place the forearms on the floor in front of you.

C. Keep the elbows stationary at the shoulders' distance or more apart.

D. Clasp the hands, interlocking the fingers to form the apex of a triangle with the elbows. Now you have the base for your headstand.

E. Place the top of your head on the floor, allowing the crown of the head to rest in the cupped hands.

F. Raise the buttocks, keeping the legs straight.

G. Slowly "walk" toward the body, still keeping the knees straight.

H. Then bring the feet off the floor, and bend the knees for balance.

I. Once you have found the balance point, continue to raise the legs into a vertical position.

J. Do not tense the body, but rest on its structural frame, completely relaxed.

K. Breathe through the nose fully and evenly.

Remain in the headstand for 1-2 minutes or longer.

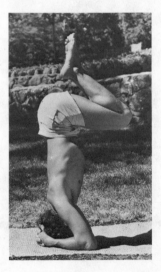

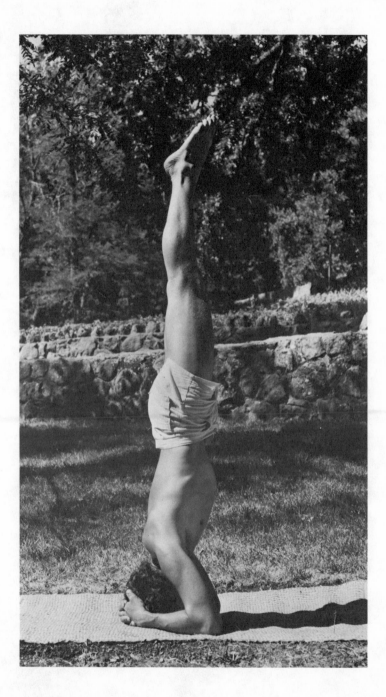

Dead Pose

Follow this period of conscious exercise with a period of conscious, deeply felt rest (see Dead Pose, page 132) to equalize the feeling of body, breath, and mind.

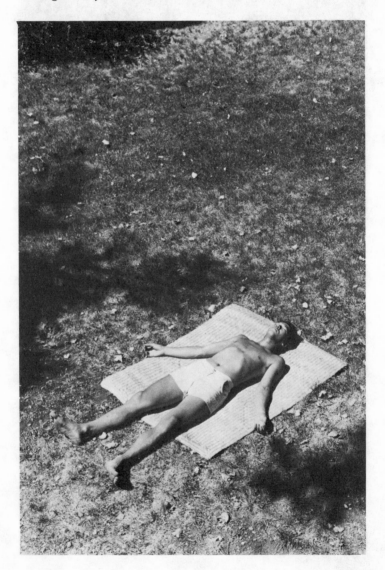

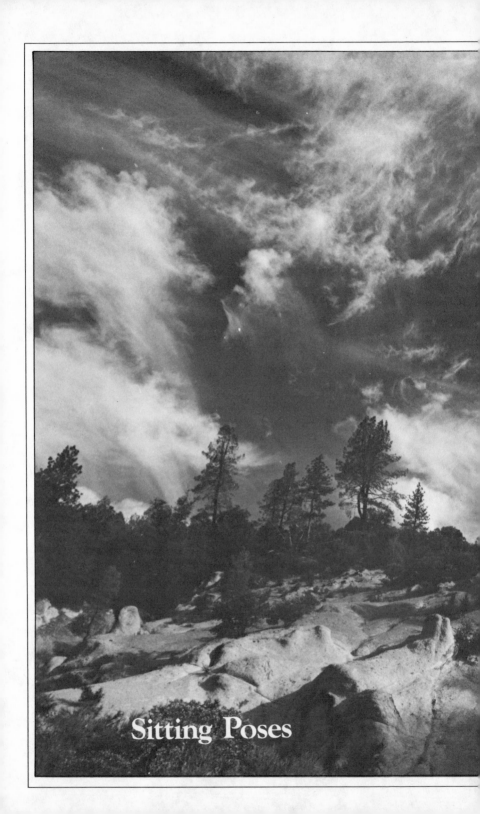

Sitting Poses

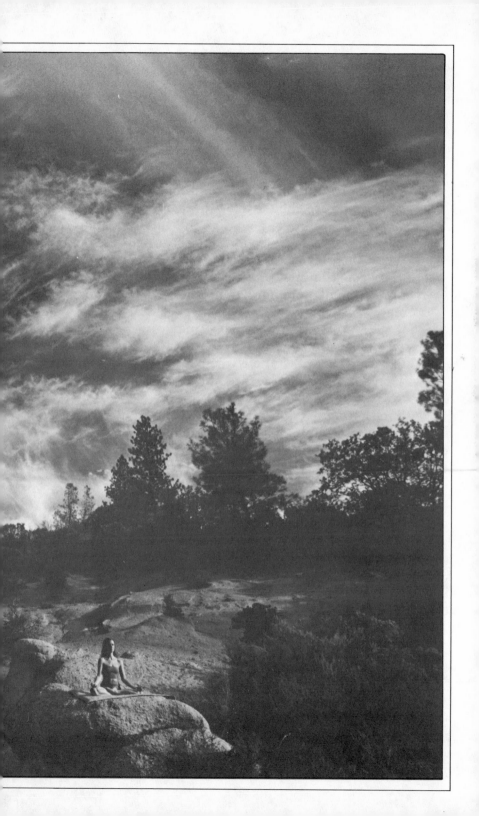

Sitting Poses for Sedentary Work, Repose, and Meditation

Anyone involved in a genuinely spiritual practice of life must sooner or later take up disciplines for formal meditation or consideration in repose. One's sitting posture should allow deep relaxation of the whole body and conservation and intensification of etheric energy flows, so that the conscious being may enjoy little or no distraction by the conventional body-consciousness and distracted awareness of the environment common to activities in the waking state.

The poses described below may also be used by anyone at any time of repose, or the relative repose of sedentary work. Those who adapt to these postures soon discover that they are in fact the most comfortable and enjoyable way to sit and be refreshed. Such sitting not only allows us to relax in a balanced condition, but it enables us, through conservation of feeling-attention, to be clarified in mind and energized with life-energy.

The Lotus Pose

A. Sit on the floor or a low platform, on top of a natural rug, pad, or thin cushion, with the legs outstretched in front of you.

B. Keeping the left leg straight, bend the right leg at the knee and grasp the right foot, placing it high up on the left thigh with the sole of the foot facing up.

C. Grasp the left foot and bring it over the right leg so it rests high up on the right thigh. The higher the crossed legs come to the mid-section, the more perfect the pose. In the perfect Lotus, both knees rest comfortably on the floor.

D. The head, chest, and spine should be kept erect, and the whole body should be made to conform to the pattern described in chapter two.

E. The relative position of the legs may be reversed, depending on your comfort. Do not, however, rest one ankle bone on top of the other.

F. Fold the hands in the lap, or place them on the knees, palms up and receptive, with the thumbs and forefingers touching.

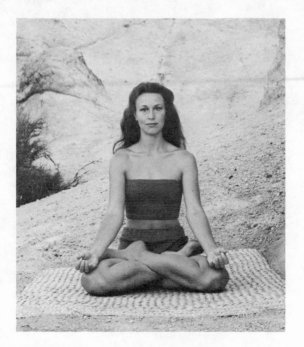

The Lotus Pose is generally considered to be the most perfect posture, not only for meditation but for any kind of sitting. It closes all the open terminals of life-force in the body and allows the energy to be continuously conducted rather than dissipated. Thus, sitting in the Lotus Pose is a means for psycho-physical refreshment, or rejuvenation. This pose is especially recommended for meditation, but you should sit in this way for meditation only when you have become proficient, and thus able to relax in the pose for prolonged periods. Sitting in a painful Lotus Pose during meditation only distracts you from your spiritual disciplines, so you should practice to become proficient in this pose as a discipline apart from meditation. All who meditate or who are preparing themselves for the discipline of meditation should practice the Lotus Pose daily, during ordinary occupations, until they can maintain it comfortably for at least half an hour to an hour.

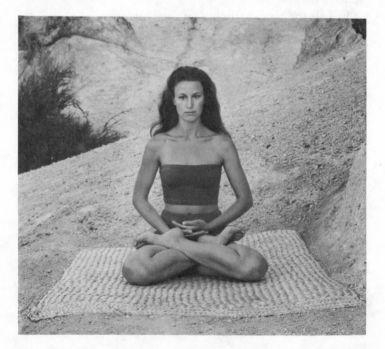

NOTE: In all references to the placement of the hands in sitting poses and the like we include the general recommendation to place them palms up and with a feeling of receptivity. When the hands are placed in the lap, this should invariably be the practice. There may, however, be occasions when — if the hands are placed on the knees or thighs — you prefer to turn them palms down and in solid contact with the body. At such times the feeling is generally one of balanced strength. You should, however, generally keep the circuit of energy in each hand closed, by touching the thumb and index finger. Other "mudras" or hand positions may be urged spontaneously in meditation, but the ones just described represent the general disposition of the hands and are common and appropriate to most occasions.

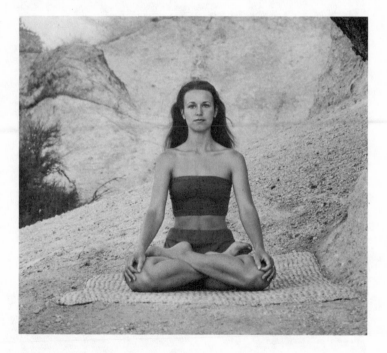

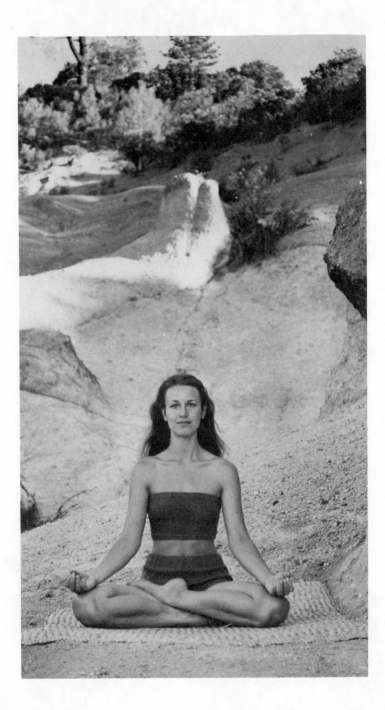

The Half-Lotus Pose

A. Sit on a covered floor or low platform with the legs extended straight out in front of you.

B. Bend the left leg at the knee and place the heel of the left foot comfortably under the perineum, the muscular area between the sex organs and the anus.

C. Keeping the left foot in this position, bend the right leg over the left so that the heel of the right foot is resting over the region of the groin. (The positions of the legs may be reversed, depending on your comfort.)

D. Do not rest the ankle bones on top of one another.

E. Fold the hands in the lap, or place them on the knees, palms up and receptive, with the thumbs and forefingers touching.

F. Keep the head and spine straight, and maintain the body as described in chapter two.

Variation:

As an alternative, the first foot may be placed under the opposite thigh, rather than the perineum, and the second foot may then rest over the opposite calf and thigh. In this position, the stretch or extension of the knees is less severe than is the case in the application of the pose as it is originally described above.

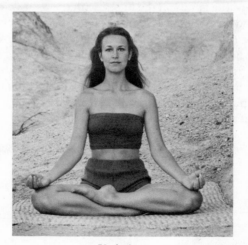

Variation

The Gentle Pose

A. Sit on a covered floor or low platform.

B. Place the soles of the feet together, sole to sole, directly in front of the body (not extended out from the thighs), knees pointing in opposite directions.

C. Grasp the toes with both hands and press both knees toward the floor, bringing the heels as close to the groin as possible.

D. With the hands on the knees, swing the body up so that the perineum rests on or close to the heels.

E. Lean slightly forward, pelvis tucked forward and up, to maintain your balance.

F. Place the hands on the knees, with the palms either facing down and firmly planted on the knees or else facing up and receptive (with thumbs and forefingers touching). The hands may also be folded in your lap.

G. A firm downward pressure may be exerted against the knees by the palms or backs of the hands. This will intensify the upward pulling sense of pressure in the midst of the lower pelvic region, at and above the perineum.

H. Breathe in the reception-release pattern.

The pose is very energizing in its effect on the whole body.

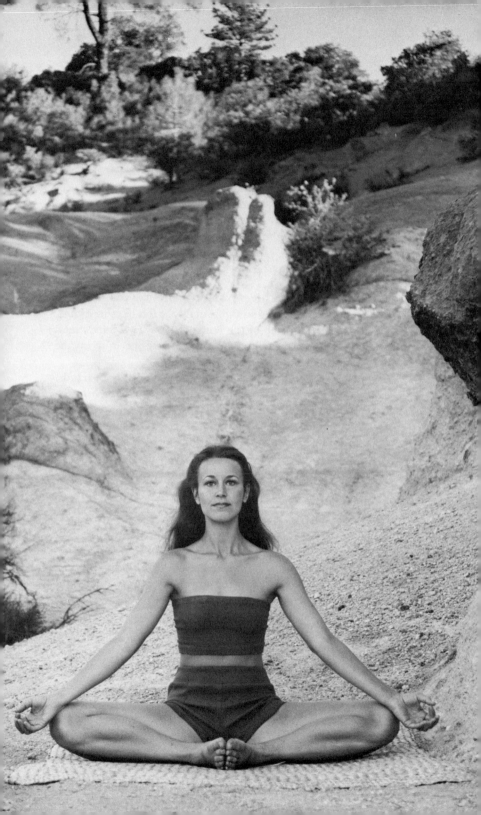

Preparing the Body for the Lotus and Other Sitting Poses

To sit comfortably in the Lotus Pose for long periods, you must stretch and elongate the ligaments in the knees. In ordinary daily activity these ligaments usually remain shortened, since the knee is kept straight or only slightly bent most of the time. Stretch these ligaments by doing the following easy exercises at random throughout each day, always being careful not to strain the body:

1. Knees to floor:

A. Sit on the floor, with legs extended in front of you.

B. Keeping the right leg straight, bend the left leg at the knee, grasp the toes and instep of the left foot with both hands, and pull that foot toward the body, so that it rests high up on the thigh of the right leg.

C. Still holding the foot on the right thigh with both hands, press the left knee to the floor. You will feel the stretch in the ligaments of the knee and the thigh.

D. Do not bounce the knee repetitively against the floor, but press and hold it there for 30 seconds or more, or as long as you can.

E. Return to the original position slowly and do the exercise with the right leg.

2. Toes to shoulders:

A. Sit on the floor with legs extended in front of you.

B. Bending the left knee, grasp the toes and instep of the left foot with both hands and pull the leg toward the body, this time raising the foot and leg into the air as if to touch the right shoulder with the left foot.

C. Hold the foot with both hands as high and as close to the body as possible, and stretch the knee toward the floor, elongating the ligaments of the knee and the muscles of the thigh.

D. Hold this position for 30 seconds or more, or as long as you can.

E. Return to the original position and repeat the exercise with the right leg.

3. Knees to floor and heels to groin (This stretching exercise is similar to the Gentle Pose, page 182):

A. Sit on the floor.

B. Place the soles of the feet together, sole to sole, in front of the body, knees pointing in opposite directions.

C. Grasp the toes with both hands and press both knees toward the floor, bringing your heels as close to the perineum as possible. You will feel the stretch in the inner thighs and groin.

D. Hold the position for 30 seconds or more. Be careful not to *strain* the ligaments and muscles, but only *stretch* them.

Other Hatha Yoga postures that help stretch the legs for the full Lotus are the Forward Stretching Pose (page 151), Position 3 of Surya Namaskar, and the Triangle or Pyramid Pose (Position 5 of Surya Namaskar). However, the best way to achieve the perfect Lotus is practice of the pose itself. Practice the stretching exercises every day and sit whenever you can, at least a few times each day, in the Lotus Pose, the Half-Lotus Pose, and the Gentle Pose.

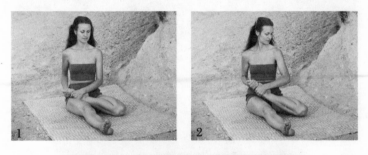

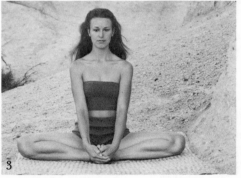

Other Sitting Postures for
Sedentary Work, Repose, and Meditation

The Diamond Pose

Some people may find that their bodies are, at least occasionally, more suited to this "Japanese-style" sitting posture.

A. Sit on the knees and calves with the buttocks resting on the insides of the feet, heels out.

B. The knees should be together, and the big toes or the balls of the feet crossed.

C. Fold the hands in the lap, or place them on the thighs, palms up and receptive, with thumb and forefinger touching.

D. Relax the body on the axes of spine and pelvis.

E. You may wish to place a small, cylindrical cushion between the calves and the thighs.

To sit in this pose for long periods also requires that the ligaments in the knees and thighs be stretched.

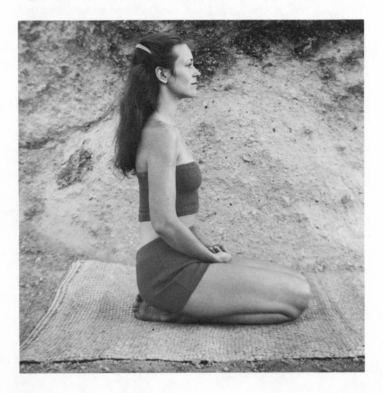

Sitting in a Chair

Until you become proficient in one or more of the recommended postures for sitting and meditation on a covered floor or low platform, you may use a chair. The chair should be firm, neither too hard nor too soft, so that the body rests well-supported from below, in an upright posture. The chair, wherever it touches the body, should be made of material that maintains room temperature, and not of metal or some similar substance. The seat or cushion should be naturally warm and of natural fiber, such as cotton or wool. To sit comfortably:

A. Assume the fundamental sitting posture we described in chapter two, with spine erect and extended, as if pulled from above, the chest high, and the pelvis horizontal to the spine, tucked easily and naturally forward and up.

B. Relax the whole body.

C. Cross the feet at the ankles and either fold the hands in the lap or rest each hand on its respective knee, palms up and receptive, with thumb and index finger touching, to conserve and conduct energy throughout the body.

D. Allow the back of the chair to support the lowest portion of the back, just below the middle of the pelvis. Do not allow the middle and upper parts of the back to rest against the chair, but maintain an upright and relaxed sitting posture.

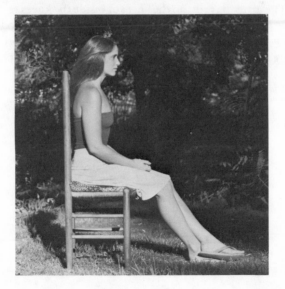

Preparing the Body for Meditation

It is also useful to prepare the body for meditation before each sitting. Along with the stretching exercises for the legs, several of the poses in the basic Hatha Yoga routine are useful for such preparation: the Downward Neck Pull (page 144), the Neck Roll (page 145), the Bow (page 148), the Plow (page 154), the Forward Bending Lotus (page 165), and the Spinal Twist (page 167).

An Alternative Position for Simple Repose

When sitting casually (not in formal meditation), a squatting pose may occasionally be found comfortable, and it is also beneficial to both the lower digestive process and the balancing of the energies above and below, in the upper and lower portions of the body.

A. Simply squat down, with the feet spread sufficiently to create a firm base for the body.

B. Allow the spine to remain as nearly vertical as possible, with the buttocks low, and the pelvis tucked slightly forward and up.

C. The arms may rest on the knees or inside the knees.

D. It is useful to occasionally rock or bounce the body, via the pelvis and buttocks, while in the squatting position — relaxing and stretching the various sections of the whole physical form.

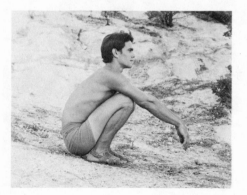

Refreshing the Body

You may also find it useful at any time of the day to refresh the body-energy consciously. There are "chakras" or centers of life-force in the hands and feet and in all the critical functional conjunctions of the body. If you are outwardly very active, you will tend to throw off energy from the vital center and the whole body in a rhythmic, fitful, and even nervous fashion. It is a process similar to orgasm, and it is performed by mental and emotional as well as physical efforts and reactivity. If you stand or walk or work with your hands a great deal, you will tend to lose energy through the feet and hands, and to tire easily. If you have to talk a lot, you will tend to lose energy through the mouth and throat and chest, and if you have to think a lot, you will tend to forget to breathe and to feel with the whole body, thus effectively "starving" the body of life-force. By consciously breathing the life-energy while keeping the body terminals closed for only a few minutes in the Lotus Pose, the Dead Pose, or one of the other Hatha Yoga poses (particularly those that involve stretching of the spine, neck, and legs), you can revitalize and refresh the whole body, restoring and circulating the force of life.

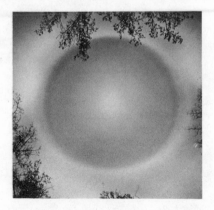

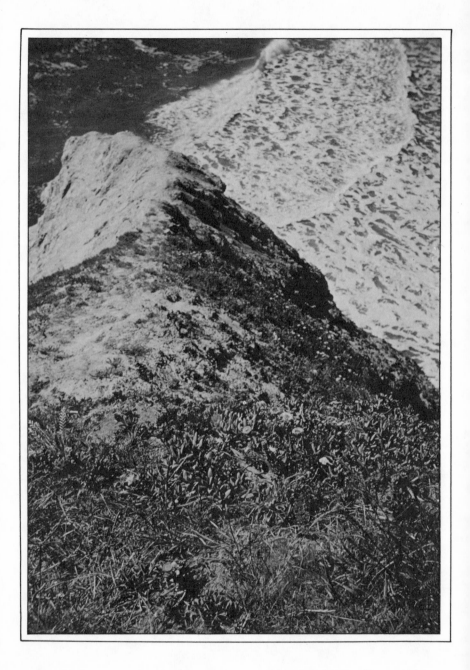

4

**The Weather System of the Life Sun:
Pranayama,
the Control of Life in Breath**

The relations between body and breath and emotion and mind and experience and environments are inherently magical, a symphony of simultaneous and mutual causes, and the devotee may become sympathetically attuned to the profusion of magical possibilities, but the Way of Divine Ignorance, or Devotional Sacrifice, is the Way of release from all conditional fascinations and obligations.

There is no objection to ordinary, disciplined, and self-surrendered application of truly Lawful principles in the conventional round of living. Such principles are expressions of whole-body orientation, in which neither the elemental body nor the etheric and life-force dimension nor the mental and conventionally psychic dimension of the whole body is exploited independently, as a strategic tool relative to the others. However, the way of knowledge, the craving and mediumistic disposition of magic or psychism, and the whole ritual of delusion that comes with devotion to changes rather than God must be undone in us, or we remain focused in dreaming and cannot awaken.

Bubba Free John
Breath and Name

4

Pranayama is an ancient technique for balancing, purifying, and intensifying the entire psycho-physical system by controlling the currents of the breath and life-force. The term literally means restraint or regulation (yama) of life-energy (prana).

Traditionally, the practice is an aspect of the total way of Hatha Yoga, which includes not only physical poses (asanas) but a whole life of moral and spiritual disciplines. At the beginning the practitioner must become proficient in the physical poses and established in an ordinary life of moderation and restraint. He must master disciplines relative to a pure and harmonious diet, study of holy texts, cleanliness, work, either celibacy or right use of sexuality, and energetic service to others. Only then, when his human life is purified and stabilized, does he take up the practice of pranayama. The traditional teachers have always warned that it is a dangerous practice, one that should not be engaged by those who are not strong and purified in body and mind and/or do not have personal guidance by an experienced teacher.

The reasons for such caution are not frivolous. In the traditional practice of pranayama, the breathing exercises are used to prepare the body for, and then to awaken within it, powerful etheric and mental energies. Once awakened, these energies (known as the "kundalini shakti") are to be manipulated to induce psychic and mystical experience and, thereby, effective transcendence of the usual bondage to the merely physical body and world. But for those who are unprepared or lack right guidance, these awakened energies can go out of control, even to the point of severely damaging the nervous system and causing great emotional and psychological distress.

From ancient times, yogis have known that there are three principal nerve channels (nadis) by which the life-force is distributed through the body, and that these have a direct correspondence to the circuitry of the respiratory and nervous systems. The secondary channels belong to the left (ida) and right (pingala) sides of the body, and they correspond to the patterns of breath through the left and right nostrils, respectively. These two etheric nerves also wind about the central and principal channel (sushumna), which is analogous to the spine. Pranayama balances the energies of the sides of the body and the nervous system, and intensifies the life-force throughout the body-being. "Ha-tha" means "sun-moon"; "yoga" means union, or the discipline that leads to union or equality. The "sun" side is the right side, which is associated with objectivity, extroversion, expansiveness of energy, emotional-vital force, action, and heat. The "moon" side is the left, associated with subjectivity, introversion, contraction of energy, mental force, inaction, and coolness.

Practitioners of the full Hatha Yoga (now popularly called "Kundalini Yoga") presume that the kundalini energy lies dormant in the usual man at the base of the spine, the lower terminal of the central nerve channel, sushumna nadi. The objective of their practice of pranayama is to purify and balance left and right, ida and pingala, in order to awaken and concentrate all available life-force in sushumna. When this etheric channel opens and the life-force begins to rise in it in concentrated form, powerful experiences of energy, inner vision, and subtle sound often ensue.

The practice of pranayama that Bubba Free John recommends for general use is a simple, ordinary, easeful discipline. The traditional practice is motivated toward escape, transcendence, and the attainment of happiness through extraordinary or subtle experience. But in conscious exercise, happiness itself is the discipline — at least for those who live it as part of the practice of the Way of Divine Ignorance. Happiness is always already our native enjoyment. So our practice of pranayama, as given here, has no extraordinary mystical goals. It serves to purify and balance the body and nervous system *gently and naturally,* without strain or danger to those who enjoy it. The practice itself is one in which the living body, including the nervous system, the mind or attention, and the universal life, are presently lived as a pure, or intense, and balanced condition.

Bubba Free John has already pointed out, in essays appearing earlier in this book, that the breath process is a secondary cycle that tends to control and modify the state or intuition of life, whereas the life-process, or constant feeling-intuition of the universal intensity or current of life, is the primary and unchanging core of all responsibility. It is love. Therefore, the secondary or breathing cycle is to the universal life what weather is to the sun. All weather more or less obstructs the sun, from the point of view of the earth. But, from the point of view of the sun, light is constant. Just so, we must maintain the position of the primary process, the "sun position" of love, or unobstructed feeling in all functions, actions, and relations. Then the breath cycle, the weather system of the whole body-being, may come under natural control. The formal and conscious exercise of prana-yama is coordinated and simultaneous control of life and breath, through *feeling*. It is weather control, wherein the sight of the Sun is never lost.

Emotions and Breathing, by Bubba Free John

Bubba Free John offers these observations of how our chronic, lower-reactive emotions affect the pattern of breathing, and how the process of breathing and emotion, the weather of the sun of life, may become a conscious exercise, both formally and under the ordinary conditions of life:

The three principal reactive emotions are fear, sorrow, and anger. If you observe yourself or another in moments of fear and like emotions, you will notice that the whole cycle of the breath, both inhalation and exhalation, is inhibited, as if frozen, unable to be initiated. In the case of the emotions that belong to the range of sorrow, the tendency is to gasp for inhalation, as if to receive consolation, and the exhalation is suppressed. And in the case of emotions in the range of anger, the exhaled breath of life is strong and aggressive, but the receptive phase, or inhalation, is inhibited.

In our ordinary adaptation to birth and circumstance, we tend to become more or less chronically used to living in a mood of existence, or a repetitive cycle of moods, that is reactive, negative, or depressed. This chronic condition may be read in the pattern of our breathing, in terms of how full or shallow it is, how easy or fitful, how suppressed or emphasized one or the other of its parts, how fully we are able to maintain natural, non-reactive feeling-attention to the patterns of life in body and relations, how easily we are able to deal with crisis events or pass through and beyond reactions to events, and so forth.

The breath should, in most of our moments, be full, easy, naturally open, pleasurable, and equal, relative to inhalation and exhalation, as well as equalizing relative to the necessary harmonies internal to the body and expressed in our relationships. We should constantly enjoy natural feeling-awareness (emotional and physical) of the whole feeling body, both tacitly and intentionally. Mind should be free as attention, usable to initiate or enjoy right action as well as right concentration, thought, and intuition. We should be able to respond, with full attention, feeling, breath, and body, to the events of life, but always from a priorly full disposition, and a Fullness that exceeds all possibilities that would empty or suppress us.

Of course, full realization of a natural and true pattern of breath and feeling depends on many factors, and a whole life of right responsibility in the truest spiritual sense. Diet and other habits of life are also constantly tending to determine conditions of mind, feeling, breath, and body. But the matter of breathing is a very direct sign as well as a controlling mechanism relative to the whole cycle of reactivity and reactive emotions. Therefore, if the process of breathing is consciously exercised, and we become aware of it as a constant process of energy and feeling rather than mere huffing and puffing, economization and control of emotional reactivity will become more and more natural to us in daily life.

The conscious exercise of breathing, or "pranayama," described in this chapter is, like conscious exercise of the body in action, as described earlier, intended to represent a general functional pattern for living moment to moment. It is also intended to represent or communicate a specific formal pattern for daily practice, that may be useful to readapt the habits of our previous living. It is important to remember that the conscious exercise of the breath should be done with full and constant *attention* and *feeling,* not frivolously and as a merely physical exercise. Only if done as an exercise of feeling-attention relative to the process of the conjunction of the body and the life-force is it true and effective.

The *process* of breathing is the object to be engaged and observed with constant feeling-attention in this exercise. It is not that we are to *watch* the breath itself, independently, but we are to participate consciously in the whole process in which we are present. Thus, the process of the whole body's breathing and living is to be felt and engaged with complete attention in this way of exercise. Then the mind will not wander through its files, and the very present matter or Truth that is always before us and at stake, and which is senior even to breath itself, will also be capable of consideration.

The Basic Form of Pranayama

As taught by Bubba Free John, the basic practice of pranayama is simply an intensified version of the process or cycle of reception-release, infilling the whole body with the universal breath of life and emptying it of all inharmonies, imbalances, toxic obstructions, and dis-eased physical and psychic, or emotional-mental, conditions. There are a few uncomplicated procedures that aid this process, but they should not become fetishistic or self-involving preoccupations for you, any more than should the practice itself.

Environment and Posture: Find a quiet place where you will not be disturbed. Pranayama can be done outdoors, if there is privacy, or else indoors, but near an open window or other source of fresh air. Practice pranayama at a time when you are already relaxed and full of energy—we recommend the period just after the Hatha Yoga poses in the late afternoon or early evening, after completing the Dead Pose. Generally, you should practice pranayama on an empty stomach, and never less than an hour after a meal (so that circulation is general to the body and not concentrated in digestion at the stomach).

Sit in one of the meditation postures, if possible. Use a cushion or mat, if you like, preferably of natural, non-synthetic materials, since these best conduct the living energy that pervades the body, the environment, and the atmosphere. The tongue should rest on the hard palate just behind the front teeth. (This is an important aspect of your posture, not only in the practice of pranayama but at all other times, because the tongue is the principal conduit of life-force between the region of the midbrain and nose and the regions of the throat and lower portions of the body.) Unless they are being used in the alternative exercises of pranayama, the hands should rest folded in the lap, or else on each respective knee, palms up and receptive, with thumbs and index fingers touching, to close the circuits of energy. Maintain an upright, stable, and relaxed sitting posture throughout the exercise.

The basic and beginning practice Bubba Free John recommends to all is extremely simple. It does not even require manipulation of the channels of the breath through single nostrils, but only simple, balanced or equal breathing through both nostrils, in time with each phase of the cycle of the breath.

Inhalation: Feel that you are gazing into and resting in a field of all-pervading life-energy. Now slowly take as much air into the lungs, and as much of this life-force into the whole body, as you possibly and comfortably can. Do not strain or force the breath beyond your capacity. The chin should be slightly lowered, so that the windpipe is opened and the passage of air and life-force is directed against the back of the throat, which should be felt to be relaxed and fully opened. The slow intake of breath should make a "rasping" sound against the back of the throat. This practice stimulates the chakra or energy-plexus at the throat, which is the seat of the life-force for the trunk and lower body. Breathe from the heart to the vital center below, with feeling, full emotional and physical feeling of the whole body.

Do not be concerned about upward or downward energy currents in the body, but simply become full, as if the whole body, visible and invisible, head to toe, is like a balloon. You should notice that, as the breath moves naturally to the vital center, it presses first upon the region of the solar plexus, then swells out the whole lower abdomen, and then fills the entire body, above and below, from the throat to the perineum, finally permeating even the head and legs and feet with vibrant force. Completely relax, opening the entire body to the intensity of unlimited energy.

As you come to the end of the inhalation, you may wish to close your eyes briefly. Hold the inhalation for just a few seconds before you begin to exhale. Do not attempt to prolong this retention; do not strain yourself in any way. You will simply find it natural and enjoyable to pause between the two phases of the cycle of breathing.

Exhalation: As you start to exhale, open your eyes again. Through both nostrils, release all the air that you have brought into the body. Like the inhalation, the exhalation should be slow and deliberate, not ragged, nervous, or forced. (Exhaling too quickly may tend to throw off life-force, nullifying the effects of the exercise.) Feel that you are eliminating not only biochemical waste by physically emptying the lungs, but also psycho-physical wastes: negative thoughts, constricted bodily feelings, unhappy emotions, and disease.

As you are completing the exhalation, allow the stomach cavity to be drawn in slightly, to help expel all the air that you inhaled. Exhale for a period about as long as you inhaled, and exhale about as much breath content as you inhaled. Then pause for an instant before beginning the next cycle of the breath.

The breathing cycle should be slow, deliberate, conscious, and full. Don't think and daydream. Your whole attention should be on feeling the process of breath and body. You should *feel* and *follow* the process fully, at every stage. And you should be sensitive to the rhythm of each cycle, so that the time and fullness of each exhalation *equals* the time and fullness of each inhalation. You should feel the whole process as a cycle of equals or balances—in and out, left and right—in which the whole body is engaged with feeling.

Repeat this cycle of pranayama again and again, for ten to fifteen minutes, during one sitting each day.

The traditional yogic practice of pranayama involves increasingly long periods of retention of breath, either in or out, after both inhalation and exhalation, and also increasingly long periods of practice, so that after several months the practitioner is engaged in pranayama for an hour or more each day. But such strenuous and forceful practice is not recommended for general practice, and it is unnecessary in any case for those who practice with the already free, feeling point of view of "conscious exercise" under all conditions of daily living.

Alternative and Advanced Versions of Simple Pranayama

After you have become proficient in the basic practice, we recommend that you alternate it, in different sittings, with the following two variations.

The first alternative variation uses only one nostril at a time upon *exhalation*. For opening and closing the nostrils, use the thumb and any other finger of either hand. The thumb and the ring finger of the right hand are traditionally used for this purpose, the index and middle fingers being folded into the palm, but you should use whichever hand and fingers feel most comfortable and natural for you. The opposite hand should rest either in the lap or on the respective knee.

To begin the practice, inhale slowly through both nostrils as instructed above. When you have completed the inhalation, close both nostrils, pause for a few seconds, and then breathe out slowly, but only through one nostril. Use only that nostril for exhalation during the first five to seven and one-half minutes of the sitting, and then finish your exercise using only the other for another and equal period of time of five to seven and one-half minutes.

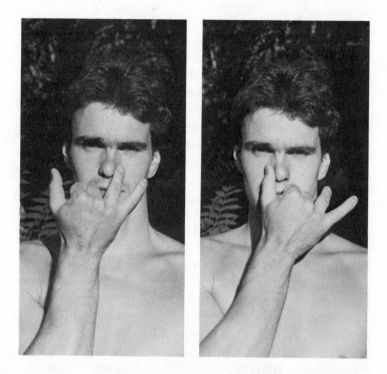

The second alternative variation involves alternate breathing, through one nostril and then the other, for each cycle of exhalation and inhalation. To begin, close the left nostril and inhale through the right side only. Then close the right nostril, pause, and then release the left nostril and exhale through it. Close both nostrils briefly. Then breathe in again through the left nostril. Remember, exercise of left and right (as well as the number of inhalations and exhalations) should be equal. And full attention, or feeling-attention, should be constant relative to each cycle and through the whole period of the exercise. Alternate again on exhalation, and so forth, for a total of ten to fifteen minutes.

Work both sides, as well as the period, number and fullness of inhalations and exhalations, equally—

with full feeling and attention throughout the exercise. Make sure to finish the exercise by exhaling through the same side with which you first inhaled, so that you have completed a full cycle of breaths through each channel of energy. In this way you maximize the balancing and harmonization of the sides, qualities, and energies of the body.

This third version of simple pranayama, or control and equalization of feeling, life-force, and breath, is the most complex, but you may also find it to be the most excellent of the three. In that case, once proficiency is attained, it may be used more or less exclusively as the daily formal exercise of pranayama. The first or basic version, however, is the form suited for random or informal application from time to time throughout the day—since it is simply a matter of conscious breathing of the life-force, with feeling, in complete, full, and balanced cycles.

After you have finished any session of formal pranayama, remain seated for a while and enjoy the natural ease and lightness you may feel. Do not rise quickly to go about your business, but relax and reintegrate yourself slowly and smoothly into the ordinary round of daily affairs of action and speech and contact with others.

Establishing Whole Body Balance Through the Exercise of Feeling-Attention, by Bubba Free John

The most significant factor in the conscious exercise of pranayama is, as in all forms of conscious exercise, the stabilization of whole body feeling-attention, or a condition that is radiating rather than contracting. The exercise itself is to be performed on the basis of a prior sense that the energy of life is full, constant, and all-pervading, regardless of the present state of relative fullness or emptiness sensed experientially and secondarily relative to the phasing of the breath. This prior sense is, at first, simply a matter of granting feeling-attention to the whole body and its relations, or of feeling-radiating as the whole body, rather than merely thinking, reacting, being inward and feeling-less, mechanical, lifeless, and self-indulgent and addicted to compulsive actions of the kind that are generated by us when we live in a chronic sense of being without pleasure. In the case of devotees, this free feeling-attention later matures into the native Fullness of Communion with the Divine Presence.

An important aspect of this particular exercise of feeling-attention, called "pranayama," or life-control, is the balancing of the two energy tendencies of the body-being. Inhalation, in general, represents the tendency of contraction, or centering, because it is a motion toward the body, or infilling. Exhalation, in general, represents the expansive, relational tendency. In the usual man or woman, adapted as we are to experience itself rather than the Condition and the Principles that precede all experiences (just as energy precedes the phasing of the breath), the tendency toward contraction becomes more or less exclusive and overwhelming. Thus, our adaptation leads to self-possession and possession by the illusions of subjectivity. The breath pattern reflects this, in that we tend to inhale with emphasis, at least fitfully or occasionally, but we tend also to exhale weakly. Therefore, even inhalation tends, in general, to be shallow, since the lungs are not properly emptied. Likewise, we generally manifest a low-grade level of feeling, which becomes dramatic only when we are reacting negatively. And we think obsessively, so that there is little free attention available for our relations or for Communion with the Reality in which we are appearing.

Through conscious exercise of pranayama, sensitivity to this dilemma may increase and some control or responsibility relative to the whole affair may begin to appear. Thus, it may be observed in practice, as we consciously require the feeling-breathing cycle to become more full and complete during both inhalation and exhalation, that there are these tendencies toward shallow breathing, scattering of attention, withdrawal of feeling—and a hunger to be filled with life, but a lack of interest or intention relative to the responsibility to communicate life. But as feeling-attention stabilizes, these tendencies also are diminished. Likewise, the tendency toward weak exhalation, common to most people under most circumstances, will diminish as feeling moves attention into the relational pattern of life.

Because of the inequality generally evidenced in the phases of our conventional breathing pattern, as well as the natural sense that exhalation *should* be longer than inhalation, teachers of pranayama often recommend practice of a cycle wherein inhalation is drawn fully to a count of one, followed by a period of retention two or more times longer, followed by a period of exhalation that is again two or more times longer than inhalation, and followed again by a period of retention two or more times as long as the inhalation. The emphasis in such routines of practice is on full inhalation, followed by prolonged retention and long, slow, full exhalation. Thus, the routine is as a purifying and balancing technique, an attempt to correct the tendency toward shallow breathing, emptiness, and weakness or unconsciousness relative to exhalation. The fundamental goal of the practice, however, is purification and, above all, mutual balance of the two phases of the breathing cycle.

In the practice recommended for general use in the present book, the same balance is contained in the form of the discipline itself—in the simple demand to breathe each phase of the cycle fully, equally, *and with feeling.* Thus, the responsibility for the balance is placed on the power of present feeling-attention itself, rather than on the relatively mechanical effort to control the ratios between the phases of the breath. Those who become proficient in pranayama and the physical culture of Hatha Yoga may use the traditional ratios and elaborations of the technique, but it is also not necessary, if the core of the practice, which is free and whole body feeling-attention, is maintained as a natural and intense discipline, both in formal practice and in the natural course of every day.

The Symptoms of Purification

Like all the other practices of conscious exercise, pranayama stirs up and releases obstructed conditions and negative tendencies. Especially at the beginning of your practice, you may feel a great deal of resistance to the discipline of pranayama. You may pass through unpleasant and difficult emotional, mental, and physical states and conditions. It may be difficult to maintain feeling-attention in the exercise without distraction. You may also experience more positive, even seemingly mystical states and blisses of energy. All such experiences are only symptoms of the process of purification and balancing, signs that pranayama and all the disciplines of conscious exercise are working effectively in the case of your own body-mind. The appropriate response to all such phenomena is to release them. Exhale them, both the positive and the negative! In any case, do not become troubled or fascinated by them, but simply continue with your disciplines each day. These phenomena may or may not fall away over time, depending on your qualities altogether, but in any case they are not your concern. The fundamental discipline is always to look and feel and be and act completely happy as the whole body, no matter what experiences may arise.

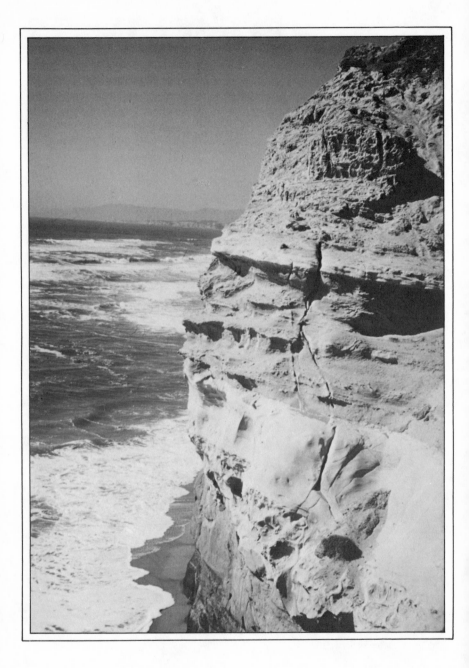

5

Exercise and the Realization of Truth

Love is more than fear, sorrow, and anger. It is not less than these. Thus, the love by which true devotees move in relationship to all beings, processes, and things is not the weak, desiring, and inward feeling-conception of the usual man or woman. It is full, it is free action, it is strong. The love which is the active principle of real spiritual life in all realms, high or low, is alive only where fear, sorrow, and anger are presently and fully encountered and transformed in the being. Love is alive only in one who is completely in touch with his or her own fear, sorrow, and anger. One who cannot permit, encounter, and face these tendencies in the contracted born-being cannot transform them at the heart. Such a one is trapped below the heart, in delusions and frustrations of body, life, emotion, sex, and all kinds of vital desiring, which make the being gravitate toward exclusion of mind in stupidity and the subconscious and unconscious conditions of awareness.

The devotee must live from the heart in Communion with the Divine Reality, and his or her living and elemental parts must come under Lawful responsibility. The being must be established in commitment to relationship, and its functions must conform to the innate economy that is Lawful in them.

Bubba Free John
The Paradox of Instruction

5

What transformations does the devotee, in the Way of Divine Ignorance, enjoy in his practice of conscious exercise? Bubba has said that, as spiritual practice proceeds beyond the reactive focusing of attention and awareness exclusively in the elemental and lower manifest levels of experience, the devotee *may* discover that he or she requires less and less overt exercise (as well as food, sexual contact, and the like) to maintain health and strength and pleasure of body and life:

> The basic postures, physical attitudes, and breathing balances, maintained as a discipline of feeling under all ordinary conditions, may become, more and more, the essence of exercise, with only random or occasional use of overt practices or games, such as Calisthenics. Even Hatha Yoga may be reduced to a few postures at random. This remark should not provide an excuse for laziness in those whose limit of experience is the waking world of gross phenomena. But those who are mature in the practice of the later stages of the Way of Divine Ignorance, or Radical Understanding, may discover that formal

bodily exercise, along with all previous obsessions in the gross plane, is less than necessary, especially as a regular and prolonged occasion. This is because a process generated prior to the gross plane or conception begins to become active in energizing, motivating, and controlling the gross being. When this higher or subtler process is stably realized, it is only necessary to maintain minimal attitudes of breath, posture, and structural availability for the natural realization of essential well-being and the ordinary fulfillment of life.

No devotee in the Way of Divine Ignorance should casually presume that such refinement of life and consciousness is true in his or her own case. Nor should any other typical individual who takes up the practice of conscious exercise. No matter how sublime your enjoyment of this practice may seem to be, simply continue with the ordinary disciplines and routines. Conscious exercise is a pleasure for the whole body, a way of yielding to open delight in the native Condition of the body itself. When your suffering has become obsolete in the fire of conscious practice, when your relationship to the Divine Presence has become so intense that *you* do not exercise, breathe, and live the body, but the Presence itself does, and when you are no longer absorbed by the gross, subjective habits that previously bound you to earthly possibilities and that made conscious exercise one of many disciplines necessary to serve your total regeneration and transformation by Grace—*then*, and only then, it may become natural and appropriate to economize your practice of this way of exercise.

Relative to "conscious exercise" as a practical extension of the discipline of God-Communion, Bubba has written:

Mind tends to concentrate, focus, objectify, differentiate, identify, name, describe, abstract, and separate. Therefore, in conscious exercise, or conscious activity under all conditions, *feel* the mind open or disperse, not as concentration but as pure attention to or contemplation of the all-pervading Reality or Presence (or, if your spiritual practice has not yet realized this Presence, simply feel the head open to space and let attention always be directed as feeling from the heart).

Likewise, the living body tends to contract, withdraw, turn in on itself, define its perimeter, enclose itself, become immune, obsessed, weak, offensive, reactive, and negatively emotional in its relations. Therefore, in conscious exercise, or conscious activity under all conditions, *feel* the living being open or disperse, entering into relationship or yielding into the all-pervading Reality or Presence. (If your spiritual practice has not yet realized this Presence, simply feel the being bodily and totally open to the air and life it breathes.)

When mind and the living body are consciously related to the all-pervading Presence, or relieved of their chronic reaction of concentration and contraction, the living being becomes an intuitive, feeling process prior to all concrete emotions, wherein all purification, change, and higher adaptation become natural and possible events.

The ultimate realization of conscious exercise, wherein its formal practice becomes random or unnecessary, involves a maturity similar to that which appears in real meditation. The man or woman who enjoys perfect intuitive dissolution in the Fire of

Divine Ignorance does not always appear to be meditating. Such a one may sit down and assume the apparently meditative mood and posture at random. But in fact his meditation is perfect and constant throughout all his ordinary activities.

Such effortless meditation, or Sahaj Samadhi (natural, effortless, uncaused rest in the Divine Condition), is the fruition of ceaseless discipline and many intense sittings in meditation, as well as a whole life of sacrifice and devotion of the whole being to God, or the Truth of Existence. Throughout the stages of the Way of Divine Ignorance, until Intuition perfects the Sacrifice, responsible and intentional activity characterizes meditation and all of the associated disciplines, including conscious exercise as it is taught in the present book. But the more perfectly the stream of ordinary life is realized in the Presence and Condition of God, the more that life becomes a form of continuous, graceful exercise of the whole being and, simultaneously, unending meditation or Bliss.

The Paradox of Bodily Existence, by Bubba Free John

When you are breathing, feel it, bodily and with emotion. Whatever you are *doing,* feel it altogether. Feel into all relations constantly. But whatever you are thinking or feeling *about* what you are doing or have done, feel what you *are* doing instead, and feel the breath of living.

If you are angry and too full of self-expression, inhale and receive and be vulnerable through all relations. And make sure the inhalations on the left side are full and clear. Then breathe evenly in the Happiness.

If you are sorrowful and full of self-pity, exhale, blow out the lungs, and bring energy, love, and strength into all your relations and make sure the exhalations on the right are full and clear. Then breathe evenly in the Happiness.

If you are afraid and full of doubt, breathe deeply and fully, with feeling. Breathe equally in and out, fully and clearly. Then breathe evenly in the Happiness.

And when fear, and sorrow, and anger are restored to the balance of life, the Fullness that exceeds and contains and is ever free of our illusion of separate life may come forth to claim your attention.

The elements of earth and water are associated with the organs of excretion and sexual union. They are associated with a tendency to go down and out, and are therefore linked with the physical or secondary effect of the inhaled breath.

The elements of fire and air are associated with the organs of digestion and respiration. They also move downward in the processes of the whole body, but they are principally associated with the tendency to go upward and outward. Therefore, they are linked with the physical and secondary effect of the exhaled breath.

The element of ether, however, is all-pervading and native to each of the elements. It always already pervades each organ and function of the whole body. It pervades both the inhaled and the exhaled breath. It precedes the motion toward the center and the motion toward the perimeter. Therefore, the element of ether is the primary and senior element of the gross dimension of the whole body. And we are obliged to be always already in communion with the universal etheric field in which the gross body is arising. This communion is established through whole body feeling-attention, in relationship, in action, and in the cycle of breathing. Such feeling is senior to the opposing tendencies of the two halves of the breath cycle and the two pairs of the lower elements.

The nervous system and the whole living body is both self-contained and open-ended. It is single and complete, and therefore must unify its functions. But it is ultimately without center or bounds, and must therefore be sacrificed, through complete feeling-attention, or love, in perpetual Communion with the Infinite Reality or Condition in which mind and life and body and relations appear.

The gross dimension of the whole body is made of a play of elements. Earth and water and fire and air oppose and play in rhythmic cycles. Ether is senior to all of these, and pervades them, through feeling. Above and senior to the gross elements is the subtle range, including perception of cosmic and pre-cosmic realms, and subtle elementals in play and opposition. The thinking mind is the lowest dimension of the subtle in the whole body of man. It reflects the play of gross elements, and conceives of logics of transcendence. But senior to the lower-reflecting mind is the subtle consciousness, above and prior to thought. It pervades the lower mind as ether pervades the lower elements. Therefore, the devotee must eventually turn the mind to its all-pervading subtle dimension, above and prior to thought.

But senior to the play and opposition of the subtle above and the gross below is the causal being, the blissful seat of primitive recoil and also primal intuition. Such is the deepest root of the heart, and the perfect Condition, or Heart, of the heart. It is Consciousness. It pervades the elements and the subtle ranges of mind, high and low. It is their Witness and their Condition. Through association with the gross and subtle appearances and functions of the whole body, the Consciousness is felt to be defined —a self, an ego, an independent being. The devotee must eventually penetrate the moods and acts of attention and Realize the Condition of consciousness. There must be Awakening to the Realization that Consciousness, or Ignorance-Radiance, the unqualified Bliss of simple or mere Existence, is the present, prior, unqualified and eternal Condition of the whole body, all beings, all relations, all experiences, and all realms or worlds.

The whole body is single and complete. Therefore, always receive everything, whatever the conditions. The whole body is undefined, centerless, open-ended, dependent on a pattern of relations in all directions to Infinity. Therefore, always release everything, whatever the conditions. The whole body, the whole world, all arising, high and low, to Infinity, is a Paradox of pairs in opposition and play, of contradictions demanding the logic of futility, and of an eternally present and obvious Condition which may always be Realized as Freedom and Happiness, prior to the conceived necessities of body, and mind, and self.

Find the Company of Truth. Hear the Teaching of Truth. Become intimate altogether with the One that is Truth.

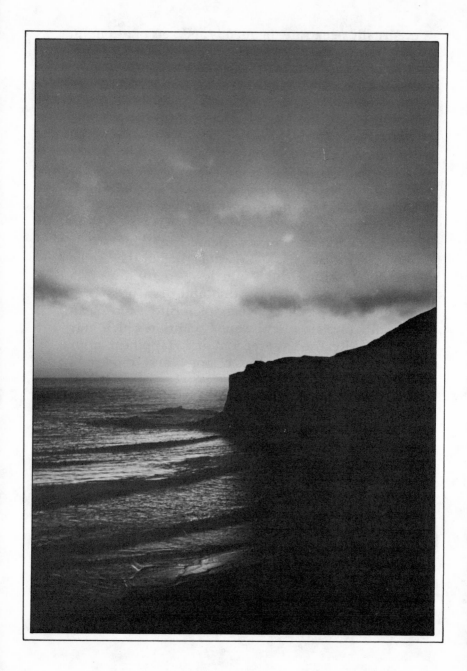

Epilogue

Light Is a Great Temptation, by Bubba Free John

Truth or God is not a Condition to be realized by willful esoteric or super-scientific efforts. Such Happiness is truly and permanently realized only on the basis of the complete moral or sacrificial transformation of the apparently individual and human consciousness. It is not a matter of merely relaxing life or body and sending the attention elsewhere by exercises of esoteric meditation. It is a matter of the undermining of the whole principle of one's ordinary and extraordinary actions and forms of knowledge.

Few are willing to endure such a process. Therefore, illusory and consoling ways have been created by compassionate, clever, and deluded men. But the scheme of all the universes, mortal and immortal, high and low, with its endless times of birth and death, and its numberless kinds of learning, is itself the way and the destiny of all ordinary and extraordinary men. Only those who weary of the usual way become willing to engage the Divine Process, in which their very life-consciousness is sacrificed in its own Condition and Nature. All others, high and low, are devoted to their own unending path, from which there is no perfect relief, except on the day all worlds, ages, and heavens dissolve in the sleep of God.

Bubba Free John
Breath and Name

Epilogue

The sun, or fascinating light, the visible vibration that can absorb us, is the principal symbol of religion and all the ways of extraordinary knowledge. The sacred practices of prophets, magicians, mystics, yogis, saints, and all ordinary believers are devoted toward knowledge of the Source Light or Creator Vibration via regressive absorption or return through the descended and progressively solid and vibratory hierarchy of manifest light. Even the various modern sciences, which pursue knowledge independent of the transformations of the experimenter and knower, may be said to be enterprises that investigate the mysteries of light, or vibratory effulgence. And, on the basis of all experiments, whether mystical or scientific, men are close to agreement on the universal concept and presumption that all appearances, forms, bodies, beings, thoughts, all events are emissions and transformations of universal and even eternal Vibratory Force or Light.

For this reason, we may say that light, or vibratory brightness, is the most universally venerated object among men. The Light of lights, seen and heard, is the principal idol to which our ways of knowing lead. To be sure, light, even most subtle or ascended, even the highest Light itself, is a great Principle of manifestation and of knowledge, but it is not Truth or very God and Reality.

Light is a great temptation. It is a mystery commonly entertained over against the idea and experience of darkness, or no-Radiance. In earlier times, life in the world was viewed as a great warfare between ascended powers of light and descended powers of darkness. And the theatre of life in the world was to be solved by a great Day, or a great impulse of Awakening, wherein those who had maintained allegiance to the highest Light would be returned, via the way of lights, to the domain of Light, above and beyond this world. And those who had been firmly committed to darkness would be excluded from Light, perhaps forever, in the domains of darkness, even the absolute Darkness below this world.

There is still an ultimate, factual, and temporal correspondence between such ideas and the theatre of universal physics. That correspondence has been all but forgotten in the cult of modern scientism, which excludes pre-scientific presumptions the way early church councils excluded the "heretical" wisdom of the ancient world. That wisdom which flourished in lights for eons remains latent in all men, even if it is now repressed by the dogmas of official experience. And that wisdom is returning now, reawakened through the service of those in whom the benighted popular and official consciousness is only superficial in its blinding effect. Even so, for those who are awakened to the super-physics of all light, Truth, the very Reality, which is salvation or Happiness, is not itself Light or any light in the exclusive sense. Light itself is ultimately resolved in a Principle that includes and is prior to both light and darkness. The Truth of life is not the victory of light over darkness. The Truth of life is not its physics of manifestation, or any kind of experiential destiny. The Truth of life is Unqualified, prior to all distinctions. It is not realized via the way of the knowledge of lights, or in the objective Shine and Sound of ultimate Brightness. It is intuited via the Wound or Mystery of Paradox, the irreducible profundity of absolute Ignorance. One whose enjoyment is Truth is thus free of all complications, even all the changes that appear in the manifesting Light. Such a one is eternally purified by the Realization that, no matter what arises, high or low, bright or dark, he does not know what even a single thing *is*.

This having been said, it is appropriate to consider what is the proper relationship between the practice of conscious exercise (or even all conscious activity) and the direct or progressive knowledge of the subtle, transcendental Sun or Light. In the older cultures, the visible sun and its light were and are worshipped and concentrated upon for the sake of physical, mental, psychic, and spiritual transformation. As such, the sun is viewed as a kind of icon, a living symbol in the universe for the Divine Sun or Prior Light that is Creative relative to the world. However, such practices, as well as their more esoteric counterparts, which conceive of the Sun within and subtly above for the same purpose, are expressions of a view of the world and of conscious existence in which Light (the Sun itself) is acknowledged as Truth and its emanations (sunlight) exploited as a method or way to Truth.

I do not propose that those who do conscious exercise use or seek the symbol of Light in this way. Although the Principle of Light may be senior to the Principle of Life, it is itself secondary to the Principle of the Awareness of both Life and Light. And all three of these Principles, which together form the foundation of every kind of esoteric and extraordinary knowledge, are fundamentals of the World-Process. They are not identical to Truth, or the Real, which has no description and is not an extension of the world, or any convention of knowledge, high or low.

What I am saying, then, is that all experience is conditional, temporary, or dependent on other conditions and Conditions. Therefore, conscious exercise is, like all ordinary experience, to be realized in Truth in the present, rather than exploited as a strategic way of attaining eventual knowledge. Conscious exercise is an ordinary discipline, founded in prior Fullness or Happiness, not an extraordinary strategy, founded in separation and distress. The discipline of conscious exercise may be realized as a direct extension of a Great Process of spiritual participation and realization in Truth. It may then be felt-intuited in terms of the whole affair of Divine Ignorance, Radical Understanding, and the spiritual Conductivity of Radiance, as these have been described in the literature of Vision Mound Ceremony.[1] But in that case, the process of conscious exercise, along with all the rest of a human life, must have matured in the midst of the radical spiritual practice of the Way of Divine Ignorance.

To take up the process of conscious exercise as an extraordinary esoteric practice from the beginning is to take on the condition of a seeker in dilemma, and to manipulate one's life by means of an idolater's idea of Light. Therefore, let the formal practice of exercise always correspond to the general level of technical participation for which you are otherwise and properly responsible as a devotee.

I urge you to begin by doing exercise, even all your activities, as an ordinary functional discipline. The exercises, as they are described in this book, are a

---

1. For a proper comprehension of the Teaching implied in this essay, you should study *The Paradox of Instruction* and *Breath and Name*, by Bubba Free John.

simple, natural, and homely practice. You are not instructed to perform the exercises as an esoteric method from the beginning, before your own experience, knowledge, and intuition combine to make you presently or already responsible for "secrets."[2] Do the exercises in ordinary ways. When you exercise, concentrate through the whole process of breathing. Feel the breath itself as pervasive energy, a living food. Engage the living breath in a natural process, in which you become filled with life on inhalation and by which you permeate and purify the living world (including your own body, mind, and psyche) on exhalation. This use of the breath in conscious exercise is fundamental, but it is not extraordinarily esoteric. It involves a natural, ordinary kind of observation and responsibility relative to the complex organism or whole body in which we appear. By means of the ordinary and conscious exercise of the body in cooperation with the living breath, or the power of feeling, established by the concentration of the conscious mind, or free attention, on the whole process, the whole game of functional activity is presently and naturally aligned or harmonized with its laws and sources.

Body, the feeling breath, and mind are each and all identical to (not other than) energy or life-force. Through conscious exercise, or conscious activity in

---

2. New devotees in the Way of Divine Communion should do the exercises in an ordinary, natural way. Those who have adapted to the "Breath of God" should exercise and live as that process implies. Those who are mature in the second stage of practice in the Way of Relational Enquiry should exercise and live in the form of true conductivity. Those involved in the Way of Re-cognition should modify their practice of conscious exercise in accordance with the technical responsibilities given them at that stage. Those in the Way of Radical Intuition should participate in all things, including conscious exercise, to the degree and in the manner that seems to be appropriate in the present moment. As the responsibilities of spiritual life increase, so should the practice of exercise be modified according to the technical form of one's general practice.

general, we affirm the lawful and functional relationship between body, feeling, breath, mind, and life-force. In the random and conventional activities of men, these agencies or dimensions of human life tend to be abused, divided, and depressed, each exploited separately, as if they were each a something apart from the others. In conscious exercise, and conscious life in general, they are enacted as a single process of mutually dependent functions. As such, they do not point to themselves or lead to meditation on their own content, but point toward their implied Law and creative Source. The Law of life is sacrifice, or unqualified relationship, and the instrumental Source of life is the Transcendental Sun or Light, the Vibratory Radiance or Current felt to permeate body, mind, and world with its all-pervading Presence, Spirit, or Breath. The Truth or Condition of life is prior to all experiential realizations of the Law and the Light. Therefore, those who would live or "exercise" consciously must also become devotees in Truth, or else their own experience will bind them.

If an individual does conscious exercise as part of a total life of spiritual practice, under the appropriate conditions communicated in the Teaching and in the Company of the Spiritual Master, he or she will, in time, simply begin to observe that the life-force, the mind, attention, the breath, all feeling, and the body at present exist as conditions of that Light which is also expressed and intuited as an all-pervading Presence. For such a one, conscious life, including conscious exercise, becomes a process of participation in the prior Condition of that Light, through conscious breathing of the Force of the Presence, and conversion or sacrifice of psycho-physical (mind-body) conditions in a cycle of reception and release. Such a one naturally and spontaneously begins to live as sacrifice, a process of transformation of life-conditions in which not self but the Divine is the Subject and the Reality. Such a one, for whom the principle of spiritual practice is conscious or intuitive sacrifice rather than accumulation of experience, also comes at last, in the maturity of the higher stages of this Way, to realize the secondary and dependent nature of the realized Light itself, and sacrifices even the Play of Light and Life to the Condition in which both are dissolved in the Unspeakable Fullness of Unqualified Reality, the Heart, the very Divine, or Real Consciousness.

Therefore, the practical principle of the esoteric realization of life is not a strategy of believing or seeking toward realization by experience. The practice, in Truth, is and must necessarily be generated by the prior Realization of Truth. The burden of such Realization is not on exercise as an esoteric method, or any other technique of knowledge, but on the Grace of the Divine itself, which always shows itself to a man or woman when he or she becomes active in the Principle of Ignorance, or prior Consciousness.

You should observe that not only are the exercises in this book described in ordinary, functional terms, but they are few in number, simple in conception, and free of strategic orientation toward the solution of any psycho-physical problem. Conscious exercise is not adapted to any goal-oriented point of view. (Just so, truly conscious human life, although it may commonly function in the conventional pattern of problems and solutions, is not fundamentally identical to any dilemma or problem orientation.) The descriptions of formal exercise in this book have been deliberately kept simple, free of the whole feeling of a grand technical or therapeutic system. The key to conscious exercise is not the exhaustive management of all kinds of technical processes, but the present realization and functional establishment of a right and feeling relationship to the fundamental and simple process of conscious life. One who does conscious exercise is actively concentrated upon that process itself in each moment of exercise. He does not concentrate on some problem, such as overweight, disease, or the need for objective God-Realization or mystical experience. Nor does he concentrate upon specific, isolated, and technical versions of his possible psycho-physiology. He concentrates upon the present and total activity that is the human life-process within the Paradox or Mystery of the infinite theatre of Existence. Thus, he does not, in principle, exercise in order to solve any problem. He simply lives his own process of life consciously. He may notice that apparent benefits arise secondary to this way of exercise, but the conscious element of his exercise is always one in which he turns from every problematic conception and motivation to simple attention in the natural event of his own activity.

This natural and intelligent attention of the being, from its center, the heart, the psychic or feeling root, involves conscious turning of the body, the breath, and the mind into coincidence with the cyclic reception-release process of life-energy. Body, breath, and mind are a single, mutual, cooperative process, each part of which must consciously be realized to depend on (and, ultimately, to be not other than) life-energy, or manifest light. Therefore, in the action of exercise, body, mind, and breath are functionally and always feelingly associated with the pervading energy in the form of life-force. This is done by consciously moving or posing the body, consciously concentrating the mind as free attention, and consciously breathing the breath as pervasive feeling, or non-personal life-force. Thus, body, mind, and breath are consciously concentrated on the life-principle, or energy, and the process of conscious exercise becomes exercise of the life-principle itself in a deeply felt cycle of inbreath-outbreath, reception-release, attention and movement. This is simply practice of the prior, harmonious condition of life as it is. Nothing is sought or directly gained in this process itself. But those who exercise and live thus may always be intuitively available to the communicated Grace of the Divine, which is the Spiritual Master and Condition of all.

What we identify as disease is, in general, a condition of combined toxemia, enervation, and mechanical disability, which is the manifest result of not living (exercising life) consciously, with full feeling, as an harmonious event of universal energy. No "cure," or solution to a specifically conceived problem or disease, is of ultimate significance. What must occur in every man or woman is a re-orientation to the principles, laws, real processes, and sources of his or her functional life. Each individual must be consciously turned away from the principle and process of disease, the problem, the dilemma, the motivation toward solutions, into the Principle and Process of his actual and prior Condition. This deeply felt and conscious turning is a matter of intuitive response to the Teaching of the Way of Divine Ignorance, and practical implementation of that response in the form of a whole life of conscious and appropriate practice in the Company of the Spiritual Master. All of the ordinary practices and disciplines communicated by Bubba Free John through the literature and services of Vision Mound Ceremony serve this present turning or re-orientation to the appropriate conditions and ultimate Condition of the human life-process. Thus, there is conscious application to diet, work, sexuality, celebration, study, service, and the like, as well as exercise. An apparent by-product of all this may be improved general health, gradual and even spontaneous healing, elimination of toxicity, intensification and increase of available life-force, increase in mechanical and mental ability, and so forth, but none of that is fundamental, or a specific goal of the practice. At best, if such changes appear, they are testimony to the essential correctness and lawful significance of the affair of conscious practice itself. It is in this spirit that the apparent benefits of conscious exercise should be viewed, and one who does the practice should always be mindful of his tendency to devote his total life in practice to remedial goals.

We tend to believe that action depletes energy and separates us from energy itself. Thus, we consider the relaxation of activity to be the obvious method for restoring or increasing available life-force. Carried to its extreme, this view results in "chronic relaxation," better known as laziness. In fact, enervation, or the chronic absence of energy, is not caused specifically and necessarily by activity. Enervation is served just as well by inactivity. Rather, enervation and every kind of inharmonious and low level of life-energy are caused by the failure to participate consciously and moment to moment, from the heart, in the cooperative process of body, breath, mind, and universal life-force in the all-pervading Divine Presence or Radiance. Thus, enervation is established more and more in one who is addicted to conventional and exclusive exploitation of the possibilities of either action or inaction. Enervation is the result of the failure to presume or be certain of all-pervading life. One who is addicted to action (the "rajasic" personality) does in fact always meditate on the idea that he is using up his life. And one who is addicted to inaction (the "tamasic" personality) does in fact always meditate on the idea that he is waiting for life and must not act. But one who knows his entire life is a constant process of changes that never end, and which is itself perfect intensity, even Unqualified Life, Light, Consciousness, and Reality, is always engaged in the harmonious event of conscious existence. Such is the true "sattwic" personality, who, whether relatively active or relatively inactive, is always consciously engaged in the same cooperative exercise of all his functions.

Where there is either chronic activity or chronic inactivity, there is the constant degenerative tendency toward enervation, toxemia, unconsciousness, weakness of body, mind, and psyche, and debilitation of all the subtle and gross forms of life. But where such chronic tendencies are not lived, their chronic destinies also start to become obsolete. Even so, one who takes on his life as conscious spiritual practice in response to the Teaching of the Spiritual Master never in fact realizes his life as true practice as long as he, in principle, practices in order to solve the problematic conditions of his life or life itself. But when he simply realizes the conscious and cooperative process of personal and relational life, and when he enjoys direct intuitive Communion with the Condition of all life, he also begins to observe positive transformations of his apparent conditions of existence. (And he continually sacrifices such transformations, be they healings, pleasures, or mystical experiences, into the Great Process and Condition, which is senior to them, and which is the very Reality or Truth, priorly and eternally free of all conditions.)

Therefore, exercise must be done, from the beginning and always, as a conscious, simple, ordinary, and functional discipline, apart from the whole affair of problems, methods, and goals. One who exercises and lives in this way may observe that the plan of exercises described in this book involves rhythms of *relative* activity and inactivity. But both phases are equally forms of activity, or the motion that is life. The more apparently active moments of exercise are analogous to exhalation in the breath cycle. They represent not the moment of the loss of energy, but the universal communication or release and permeation of energy, whereby the one who exercises is also and totally included. Just so, the more apparently relaxed or inactive moments of exercise are analogous to inhalation in the breath cycle. They represent not inaction or the prevention of action, but the profound action of opening, drawing upon, and receiving the all-pervasive energy or universal light. Therefore, in fact, every moment of conscious exercise is action, the motion of feeling. All such action involves the intensifying and transforming play of life-force. Energy is thus always being "restored," and body states, feeling states, breath characteristics, and conditions of thought and attention are always being transformed in every moment of conscious exercise and conscious life, independent of any problem-oriented strategy to do such things.

In the actual or formal practice of conscious exercise, there should be no daydreaming, but constant feeling-attention to coordination of body and breath in the play of life-force. There should be no laziness, but devotion or complete, deeply felt adaptation of the body to the deliberate and full display of chosen movements and poses. And there should be no dead breath, no small chemistry, but intentional and full use of breath as a feeling instrument for actual and present ingestion, translation, and transfer of felt life-energy. As such, conscious exercise becomes a paradigm for the conscious realization of the whole of life. The formal practice of conscious exercise is merely a concentrated occasion or "lesson," whereby we are instructed in the realization of every ordinary action as a conscious but non-formal exercise in the same sense. A life realized and expressed by such a discipline is always already movement in sunlight, with eyes fixed firmly on the Sun. And the devotee of Truth is not only so realized in fact, but also eternally and immeasurably free, both Night and Day.

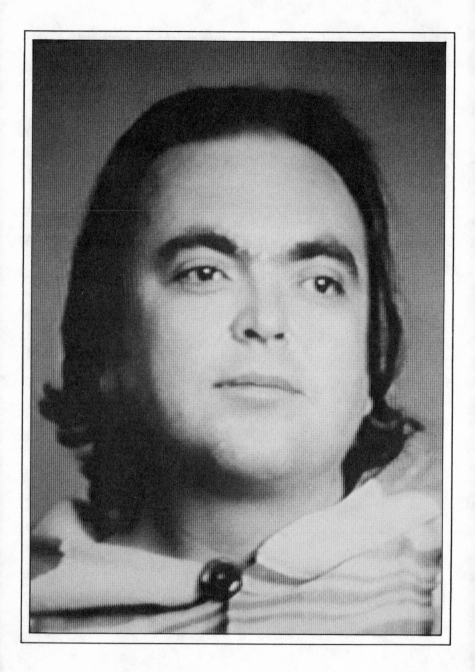

An Invitation

Spiritual Fire and
the Presence That Is God

For those who are becoming available to the process of transformation in the Divine, I have established the Way of Divine Communion, which is the simple way of loving submission and attention to God. Many will respond to my Teaching, and all are welcome to approach me through the Teaching and the services of Vision Mound Ceremony, who are simply suffering the common failures of life. To all of them I simply say, come happily, with the urge to happiness, to peace, to love, and to a better realization of your born life. The Lord of all the worlds is Radiant before you. If you will simply direct yourself to the service and awareness of the Divine, the Services of God will be given to you.

It is not necessary or even possible for you to "believe" in God or know the Character of the Divine Reality. But if you can see that you do not exist by your own creature power, and if you can begin to consider the alignment of your life with the unspeakable Source or Condition that is truly responsible for and ultimately identical to your very existence, then you can do the spiritual practice of Communion with God. I urge and welcome all who can manage such sympathy to accept the simple and pleasurable disciplines I will recommend.

For those who would thus adapt themselves, I recommend a way that is easy to conceive and fulfill. Simply turn to God. Submit, surrender yourself to God. Love and receive God. The Divine is a Presence you will come to know. That Presence is only God. If you will devote or sacrifice yourself to that all-pervading Presence, God will transform your knowledge, and you will realize only God at last.

Bubba Free John
Breath and Name

An Invitation

Conscious exercise is only one of a number of practical disciplines assumed by those who are beginning the Way of Divine Ignorance, or Radical Understanding, as taught by Bubba Free John. For your interest, we would like to describe that Way more fully—particularly its initiation and foundation stage, the Way of Divine Communion.

Devotional Practice and the Grace of the Spiritual Master

True spiritual practice in the Way of Divine Ignorance ultimately transforms the whole body and conscious being, down to the very cells. It is an inconceivable and marvelous process. But the effective principle of this Divine transmutation is not our own practice of specific disciplines. It is, rather, the practical spiritual relationship to the Spiritual Master. The true form of this relationship is not an imaginary, cultic, and merely enthusiastic affection, but a living spiritual connection, face to face and heart to heart.

All the great ancient traditions agree that such a relationship is the most wonderful and sublime opportunity for any human being. Those who do live as devotees of true Teachers treasure that spiritual link beyond all other relations and possibilities. It is the very foundation of their lives. But it is not an easy affair. Nor is it a matter of childish dependence on the part of the devotee, and parental consolation on the part of the Master. Such a relationship, rightly lived, is immensely happy and full of love, but there is nothing, in principle, gleeful or romantic about it. It rests upon our availability to the Spiritual Master's argument, which is at once a sobering criticism of the quality and consequences of our usual lives, and a radically ecstatic communication of our Condition in Truth, which is Divine. And the natural, relational practices given to the devotee by the Spiritual Master only serve to prepare body, feeling, and attention for the unspeakable re-adaptation to life in and as this Divine Reality. This preparation is not just a conventional purification and harmonization of our lives. Even from the beginning, it is a constant frustration of the self-oriented mood that we chronically generate. Its principle is the Divine Ignorance that is the very Nature of our existence, prior to our usual sense of being identified with a bodily personality and concrete experience.

If you wish to consider the argument of Divine Ignorance more fully, you must consult the source books of Bubba's Teaching, *The Paradox of Instruction* and *Breath and Name*. Here it is only necessary to say that the devotee in this Way is responsible from the beginning for an enlightened, already selfless approach to every moment of life—even as his tendencies to self-possession of every kind continue to arise. He has no right to self-possession or egoic consolation, even in the literal fulfillment of the specific disciplines, such as conscious exercise. Yet he is responsible to fulfill the disciplines, always, happily, and without relapse. Thus, his life becomes a kind of hidden asceticism in the midst of ordinary human enterprise and action. The frustration of all egoic or self-possessed tendencies becomes a purifying heat and, later, a transforming fire:

> Be applied to the Law [of sacrifice] bodily, emotionally, with present attention in relationship. Persist in the ordinary disciplines . . . and, when appropriate, the spiritual practices as well. Endure the heat. Do not indulge un-Lawful tendencies, but also do not become concerned by any tendencies you feel to persist in spite of discipline. Thus, the heat will always increase. You will be purified, transformed, and re-adapted in your adaptations. Turn your view from subjective conditions of thinking, emotional inclinations, obsessive desires, bodily states, and circumstances of conventional opportunity. Turn to the Divine in Ignorance. Allow the heat of discipline to provide a link to the Presence shown to all devotees by Grace. The heat awakened in the discipline is the power or devotional fire that then becomes the available energy of spiritual practice. Thus, spiritual discipline only follows in the case of practical discipline. The grosser elements must be transformed in fire before the subtle is revealed above. Then even the subtle must be converted and dissolved in the same fire. That fire is the Heart, the Radiance, the Condition of conditions. It is the Principle in the midst, the fire in the middle ("pyramid"), beyond both the lower and the higher physics. It is Bright in Igno-

rance. It is the Light in discipline and devotion. It is the devotee of the Presence, and it is the Presence itself.[1]

The Practical Disciplines of the First Stage of Practice

Those who are moved to take up the whole Way of life Bubba offers begin their practice with the Way of Divine Communion. Along with conscious exercise, the initial, practical, preparatory disciplines of this stage are:

☐ observance of a simple sacrament, the Celebration of Universal Sacrifice, in which the devotee gives to the Divine and receives in return a simple gift of fruit or flowers, as a tangible demonstration of the principle of his spiritual practice, which is reception-release, or mutual sacrifice;

☐ regular study of the critical and instructive Teaching of Bubba Free John, along with devotional literature from the traditions of esoteric spirituality, both privately and in groups;

☐ full-time employment in responsible, productive work or study, and maintenance of a clean, orderly, harmonious household or intimate environment;

☐ maintenance of natural health practices and moderate, naturally nutritious, lacto-vegetarian diet, avoiding traditional dietary accessories (meat, fish, eggs, poultry, alcohol, tobacco, coffee, refined and processed foods), except during occasional celebrations with intimate friends and family, entirely avoid-

---

1. *Breath and Name*, II, 5.24, pp. 105-106.

ing social drugs (marijuana, hallucinogens, and the like), and using conventional or unnatural medicinal drugs or cures only when absolutely necessary;

☐ engagement of sexual play only in the context of a lifelong commitment to a marriage relationship (legally recognized if between heterosexuals, and equally responsible and committed if between homosexuals), and only under the intense relational conditions of genuine love-desire;

☐ heart-felt and practical service to others, to the Spiritual Master, and to the Divine Reality in all circumstances and in the form of all actions.

You can find more detailed information on these disciplines in *Breath and Name,* the comprehensive source text on the whole Way of Divine Communion, and *The Eating Gorilla Comes in Peace,* which is the manual of practical instructions on diet and health practices.

Taken together, all these homely, tangible, initial disciplines provide a living spiritual practice for every waking moment. Like conscious exercise, they are all lawful, congenial, and essentially simple, turning the body, emotions, and mind out of self-possession and into the condition of relationship, or feeling sacrifice. Because we are all chronically self-oriented, however, the devotee who is mature in these practices is already an uncommon individual. The heat of practice has purified him to the degree that he no longer lives from the usual obsessed and inward-turned point of view. He continually turns into relationship. He is happy. He serves, and he loves, without necessary self-reference. All kinds of subjective inclinations and desires continue to arise in him, but he is steadily committed to a moral, responsible life of spiritual consideration and effective action. He is simply a mature human being, as man or woman.

Initiation into the Divine Presence

At this initial point of maturity in practice, the devotee may begin to enjoy the living Company of the Spiritual Master. Bubba Free John has no public life, and he rarely if ever sees those devotees who are still immature in their practice of the life-conditions described above. Moreover, he meets even with mature devotees only occasionally, most often in formal, silent, sitting meditation. The reason for these restrictions of his availability is simple—and sublime. The human Company of a true Spiritual Master is *spontaneously* initiatory; it begins to work transforming effects on all those who approach it. But only those who are practically prepared, physically, emotionally, and mentally, can make real and true use of such contact. For others, it is only fascinating or disturbing.

In the Spiritual Master's Company, the prepared devotee soon begins to enjoy one of the critical awakenings or initiations of spiritual or real life. Without effort on his own part, but through the conscious and Graceful agency of the Spiritual Master, he begins literally to feel and be absorbed in the all-pervading Presence that is God. He feels this Presence from the heart and with his whole being, undeniably. And he begins to live in this Divine Presence constantly, in daily life and in formal meditation. Thus, in one who is established in the heat of purifying discipline, the Spiritual Master ignites the fire of Divine transformation.

The religious and spiritual literatures of mankind offer innumerable descriptions of the Presence of God as a specific Energy, Image, Sound, or Light objectively perceived by the mind or ego-soul. But the true Divine Presence is a paradox, and so is the true devotee's relationship to it. He feels it tangibly, as a surrounding and all-pervading Power; and at the same time, most intimately, he feels it intuitively as his very Condition, the living Core of his being. It is not other than his own Nature and Consciousness. Therefore, it cannot be objectively perceived or experienced, and it cannot truly be described. But for the devotee who is awakened in this Presence, there is no doubt about it. The Spiritual Master lives always as the Presence itself, and he attracts the devotee into that Presence by Grace. This awakening quickens the spiritual process immeasurably.

The Spiritual Disciplines of the Way of Divine Communion

The devotee begins to contemplate and open himself to the Presence of God through two simple spiritual disciplines, the Breath of God and the Name of God.

The practice of the Breath of God is a new adaptation of the natural discipline of breathing that one learns in conscious exercise. Randomly, upon inhalation, the devotee receives the enlivening and transforming Presence, allowing it to fill his whole being, head to toe, body, emotions, and mind. And randomly with the exhalation he releases all accumulated, subjective, and contracted conditions of the being into the Presence, allowing the Presence itself to Radiate through all his functions and even the universe itself. This practice is different from his previous discipline of breathing: the Divine Presence is felt as the Source or Condition of both the devotee and the objective life-energy to which he originally aligned himself. This reception-release "between" the devotee and the Presence is profound and indescribable, and at the same time a most natural and ordinary practice.

The practice of the Name of God is not a traditional invocation or use of a mantra or sound-device, but it is, rather, direct recollection of the Presence. It is contemplation of God from the heart, not only with the mind or attention but with every particle of the whole body. At times the devotee may aid this silent recollection with the use of the verbal Name "God," but not in a methodical or repetitive way. It is simply a natural reminder, restoring him to the contemplative mood.

The devotee enjoys these disciplines most intensely in periods of formal meditation twice each day. But he also engages them randomly in the midst of ordinary activities, integrating them with his practice of the life-conditions. When he matures in this single and integral practice, he begins to behold and feed upon the Presence continually, in the midst of every kind of circumstance.

The Higher Stages of Spiritual Practice

Clearly, such a devotee is already a joyously transformed being. Eventually it becomes appropriate for him (or her) to take up the practice of the second stage of the Way of Divine Ignorance, which is the Way of Relational Enquiry, and in due time the third and fourth stages, the Way of Re-cognition and the Way of Radical Intuition. As his ordinary human life becomes more and more a matter of easeful discipline and enjoyment, the devotee becomes increasingly sensitive and available to subtler, more esoteric processes of existence. The disciplines of the higher stages, like those of the Way of Divine Communion, are natural, relational, or released expressions of the whole body happiness that is our Condition in Truth. They are disciplines of love, by which the devotee simultaneously adapts to and intuitively penetrates the illusions of higher experience and knowledge, and so comes utterly to rest in the prior and native state of man, which is Happiness itself, Divine Ignorance.

In the final stage of practice, the devotee's persistence in the discipline of unobstructed feeling-intuition has become spontaneous and absolute. Thus, like the Spiritual Master himself, he passes absolutely beyond the implications of all experience, all anxiety, every kind of birth, life, and death. At the same time, his ordinary life continues, albeit in a sublimely renewed way. This Realization is a paradox. If you wish to consider it further, you should consult *The Paradox of Instruction,* in which Bubba thoroughly describes the progression of practice, experience, and understanding in each of the advancing stages. He shows how the ultimate Enjoyment in the Way of Divine Ignorance surpasses every kind of objective or experiential vision, bliss, and illumination enjoyed and taught by the yogis, saints, and sages of all spiritual traditions.

An Invitation to Participate in the Services of Vision Mound Ceremony

Vision Mound Ceremony is the public education division of The Free Primitive Church of Divine Communion, commonly known as The Free Communion Church. These two institutional extensions of the revelatory Teaching work of Bubba Free John serve two principal and integrally related functions in the world: to communicate and to provide adequate facilities for the communication of the Teaching of Bubba Free John, and to provide, serve, and maintain his domestic living requirements as well as manage access to him for all who respond to his argument and live according to the Way of Divine Ignorance.

We invite you to consider this Teaching, and, if you are moved to the happy offenses and sacrifices it demands, to become established in a direct and transforming spiritual relationship with Bubba Free John. The appearance of the human Spiritual Master is brief, and those who resort to his Company enjoy a Graceful privilege unknown to common men and women, including the usual spiritual seeker. "Become this Sacrifice with me and rise from this death into the Condition of the Heaven-Born." This is Bubba Free John's invitation to you. Vision Mound Ceremony exists only to serve your direct approach, and that of all other devotees, to Bubba as Spiritual Master.

The editorial and educational staff of Vision Mound Ceremony is responsible for the production and dissemination of all the literature and educational media or programs necessary for the practice of the Way of Divine Ignorance. Those who are interested in that full process, of which conscious exercise is a part, should read the essential source texts of this Way. *The Paradox of Instruction: An Introduction to the Esoteric Spiritual Teaching of Bubba Free John* is the essential and summary communication of all the stages and aspects of the Way, and is to be used as the principal source text by devotees in every stage. *Breath and Name: The Initiation and Foundation Practices of Free Spiritual Life* is a manual that specifically describes the practice of the

Way of Divine Communion. It presents instructions in both the practical and the spiritual or natural responsibilities and conditions of the Divine life realized and assumed in the first stage of practice. Since, however, it is also the foundation description of the practice and process of the whole Way, it remains a principal source text for every stage. Also of primary importance to all devotees entering the Way of Divine Communion, in addition to the present book, are *The Eating Gorilla Comes in Peace,* the source book on diet and health practices, and *Love of the Two-Armed Form,* the source text on regenerative sexuality and the higher or specifically human practice of true intimacy. The instructions in these texts also remain useful throughout one's life of practice. Although the specific practices themselves simply become enjoyments that are "second nature" to one's ordinary life, the core or principle of all practices—which is love, or unobstructed feeling-attention in all relations—is communicated in a specifically useful way in each of these texts. Taken together, these five texts (including *Conscious Exercise and the Transcendental Sun*) represent a complete foundation and the ultimate vision of a truly enlightened culture of ordinary, pleasurable human existence.

The Way of Divine Ignorance is a Divine Way, founded consciously in the Divine Condition from the beginning. It is the Way of ordinary re-adaptation rather than search for extraordinary attainment, a way of dissolution rather than experience. All necessary instructions are openly given and can be easily grasped by anyone whose orientation to practice is true, and whose commitment to Bubba Free John as Spiritual Master is straightforward, real, and based in true hearing of his Teaching.

If you are interested in learning more about the

forms of personal involvement that you may enjoy with Bubba Free John as Spiritual Master, please write to:

Vision Mound Ceremony
P.O. Box 3680
Clearlake Highlands, California 95422

Vision Mound Ceremony is the public education division of The Free Primitive Church of Divine Communion, commonly known as The Free Communion Church.

Appendix

Books on the physiology, psychology, and practice of formal exercise, and other forms of physical play, which may be adapted to the practice of "conscious exercise"

The formal physical regime recommended in any of these books may be found useful as an extension of "conscious exercise." The more esoteric recommendations, such as those relating to chakras, kundalini, meditation, and so forth, illustrate the spiritual or yogic point of view behind many of the traditional approaches to health and well-being, but they should not be practiced except by those who are under guidance in a like tradition. Devotees in the Way of Divine Ignorance should simply compare these recommendations to their own given responsibilities and practice.

Vision Mound Ceremony makes many of these books available directly through the mail. For a list of titles in stock or for information to help you obtain titles we do not carry, please write to:

The Dawn Horse Book Depot
P.O. Box 3680
Clearlake Highlands, California 95422

I. The Physiology of Exercise

1. *Atlas of Human Anatomy, Simplified,* by F. Gaynor Evans. Ames, Iowa: Littlefield, Adams & Co., 1958.

2. *The Quest of Wholeness: An Evaluation of the Yoga Discipline from the Point of View of Neurophysiology* (Translation from the original Sanskrit of Patanjali's Yoga-Sutras with a critical commentary), by S. Sorenson. Reykjavik, Iceland: Prentsmidja Jons Helgasmar, 1971.

3. *Foundations of Conditioning,* by Harold B. Falls, Earl L. Wallis, and Gene A. Logan. New York: Academic Press, 1970.

4. *Physiology of Exercise, for Physical Education and Athletes,* by Herbert A. Devries. 2d ed. Dubuque, Iowa: Wm. C. Brown, 1974.

5. *Physiology and Physical Activity,* by Brian J. Sharkey, New York: Harper & Row, 1975.

6. *Kinesiology and Applied Anatomy: The Science of Human Movement,* by Philip J. Rasch and Roger K. Burke. 5th ed. Philadelphia: Lea & Febiger, 1974.

7. *Mensendieck: Your Posture and Your Pains,* by Ellen B. Lagerwerff and Karen A. Perlroth. Garden City, New York: Anchor Press/Doubleday, 1973.

8. *Human Movement Potential: Its Ideokinetic Facilitation,* by Lulu E. Sweigard. New York: Harper & Row, 1974.

9. *Body Dynamics,* by Eleanor Metheny. McGraw-Hill Series in Health Education, Physical Education, and Recreation. New York: McGraw-Hill, 1952.

10. *The Principles of Exercise Therapy,* by M. Dena Gardiner. 3d ed. London: G. Bell and Sons, 1976.

11. *The Thinking Body: A Study of the Balancing Forces of Dynamic Man,* by Mabel Elsworth Todd. New York: Dance Horizons, 1972.

II. The Philosophy and Psychology of Exercise

1a. *Energy: The Vital Polarity in the Healing Art,* by Randolph Stone. 2d ed. Originally published as *New Energy Concept of the Healing Art.* Chicago: the author, 1957.

1b. *The Wireless Anatomy of Man and Its Function,* by Randolph Stone. Chicago: the author, 1953.

2. *Awareness Through Movement: Health Exercises for Personal Growth,* by Moshe Feldenkrais. New York: Harper & Row, 1972.

3. *The Resurrection of the Body: The Writings of F. Matthias Alexander.* Selected and introduced by Edward Maisel. New York: Dell Publishing Co., 1971.

4. *The Body Has Its Reasons: Anti-Exercises and Self-Awareness,* by Therese Bertherat and Carol Bernstein. New York: Pantheon Books, 1977.

5. *Body and Mature Behavior: A Study of Anxiety, Sex, Gravitation & Learning,* by Moshe Feldenkrais. New York: International Universities Press, 1973.

6. *The Body Reveals: An Illustrated Guide to the Psychology of the Body,* by Ron Kurtz and Hector Prestera. New York: Harper & Row, 1976.

III. The Vital Center

1. *The Solar Plexus or Abdominal Brain,* by Theron Q. Dumont. Wheaton, Illinois: Yoga Publication Society, c. 1921.

2. *Hara: The Vital Centre of Man,* by Karlfried Graf von Durckheim. London: George Allen & Unwin, 1962.

3. *Ground, Round.* Mendocino, California: Moving On, 197?.

4. *Meditation Gut Enlightenment: The Way of Hara,* by Haruo Yamaoka. South San Francisco: Heian International Publishing Company, 1976.

5. *The Human Ground,* by Stanley Keleman. 2d ed. rev. from the original paper "Bioenergetic Concepts of Grounding." San Francisco: Lodestar Press, 1973.

IV. Surya Namaskar (Surya Namaskar is also treated in some of the titles listed under "Hatha Yoga")

1. *The Ten-Point Way to Health: Surya Namaskars,* by Shrimant Balasahib Pandit Pratinidhi, the Rajah of Aundh. Bombay: D. B. Taraporevala Sons, 1974.

2. *Surya Namaskar: A Technique in Solar Vitalization,* by Swami Shivananda Saraswati. Monghyr, India: Bihar School of Yoga, 1973.

3. *Surya Namaskar: An Ancient Indian Exercise,* by Bhawanrao Pant Pratinidhi (Rajah of Aundh) to his son, Apa Pant. Bombay: Orient Longmans, 1970.

V. Calisthenics and More Active Exercise

1a. *Aerobics,* by Kenneth H. Cooper. New York: Bantam Books, 1969.

1b. *The New Aerobics,* by Kenneth H. Cooper. New York: Bantam Books, 1972.

1c. *Aerobics for Women,* by Mildred Cooper and Kenneth H. Cooper. New York: Bantam Books, 1973.

2. *Royal Canadian Air Force Exercise Plans for Physical Fitness.* Rev. ed. New York: Pocket Books, 1974.

3. *The Official YMCA Physical Fitness Handbook,* by Clayton R. Myers. New York: Popular Library, 1975.

4. *Exercise!,* by Herbert M. Shelton. Chicago: Natural Hygiene Press, 1971.

5. *Total Fitness: In 30 Minutes a Week,* by Laurence E. Morehouse and Leonard Gross. New York: Pocket Books, 1976.

6. *The Way to Vibrant Health: A Manual of Bioenergetic Exercises,* by Alexander Lowen and Leslie Lowen. New York: Harper & Row, 1977.

7. *Fitness Program, with Spine Motion,* by Paul C. Bragg. Burbank, California: Health Science, 1973.

8. *The Baby Exercise Book: For the First Fifteen Months,* by Janine Levy. 2d Am. ed. New York: Random House, Pantheon Books, 1975.

VI. Hatha Yoga

1. *Science of Yoga: Commentary on Gherand Samhita.* Monghyr, India: Bihar School of Yoga, no date.

2. *The Gheranda Samhita.* Translated by Rai Bahadur Srisa Chandra Vasu. 2d ed. New Delhi: Oriental Books Reprint Corp., 1975.

3. *Yoga in Simple,* by Swami Nityananda Saraswati. Monghyr, India: International Yoga Fellowship, 1971.

4a. *Asana, Pranayama, Mudra, Bandha,* by Swami Satyananda Saraswati. double ed. Monghyr, India: Bihar School of Yoga, 1973.

4b. *Notes on Asana, Pranayama, Mudra, & Bandha.* Monghyr, India: Bihar School of Yoga, no date.

5a. *Health Benefits of Backward Bending Asanas,* by Swami Nischalananda. Monghyr, India: Bihar School of Yoga, 1974.

5b. *Health Benefits of Forward Bending Asanas,* by Swami Nischalananda. Monghyr, India: Bihar School of Yoga, 1974.

5c. *Health Benefits of Inverted Asanas,* by Swami Nischalananda Saraswati. Monghyr, India: Bihar School of Yoga, 1973.

6. *Nawa Yogini Tantra: For Every Woman Who Seeks Health, Happiness and Self-Realization,* by Swami Muktananda Saraswati. Monghyr, India: Bihar School of Yoga, 1977.

7. *The Secrets of Prana, Pranayama & Yoga-Asanas,* by Swami Narayanananda. 2d ed. rev. Rishikesh, India: Narayanananda Universal Yoga Trust, 1967.

8. *Yoga Asanas,* by Sri Swami Sivananda. 14th ed. Sivanandanagar, India: The Divine Life Society, 1969.

9. *The Complete Illustrated Book of Yoga,* by Swami Vishnudevananda. New York: The Julian Press, 1960.

10. *Yoga Asanas: A Natural Method of Physical and Mental Training,* by Louis Frederic. New York: Samuel Weiser, 1973.

11. *First Steps to Higher Yoga: An Exposition of First Five Constituents of Yoga,* by Swami Vyas Dev Ji (Swami Yogeshwaranand Saraswati). Rishikesh, India: Yoga Niketan Trust, 1970.

12. *Light on Yoga (Yoga Dipika),* by B. R. S. Iyengar. rev. ed. New York: Schocken Books, 1977.

13. *Yoga: Harmony of Body, Mind and Soul (Yoga, Yoga Therapy with Yogic Postures),* by Chandrasekhar G. Thakkur. Bombay: Yoga Research Center, Ancient Wisdom Publications, 1977.

14. *Yogic Asanas for Health and Vigour: A Physiological Exposition,* by V. G. Rele. 10th ed. Bombay: D. B. Taraporevala Sons, 1972.

15a. *Practical Yoga: A Pictorial Approach,* by Masahiro Oki. abr. ed. Tokyo: Japan Publications, 1970.

15b.*Healing Yourself Through Okido Yoga,* by Masahiro Oki. Tokyo: Japan Publications, 1977.

16. *The Yoga System of Health and Relief from Tension,* by Yogi Vithaldas. New York: Bell Publishing Company, 1957.

17a. *Yogic Therapy: Its Basic Principles and Methods,* by Swami Kuvalayananda and S. L. Vinekar. New Delhi: Ministry of Health, Government of India, 1963. Reprinted 1971.

17b.*Asanas,* by Swami Kuvalayananda. Bombay: Popular Prakashan, 1971.

18. *Easy Stretching Postures for Vitality and Beauty,* by Randolph Stone. Chicago: the author, 1954.

19. *The Five Rites of Rejuvenation (Plus One), or the Eye of Revelation,* by Peter Kelder. Vista, California: Borderland Sciences Research Foundation, 1975.

20. *Breath, Sleep, the Heart, and Life: The Revolutionary Health Yoga of Pundit Acharya.* Lower Lake, California: The Dawn Horse Press, 1975.

21. *Yoga and Health,* by Selvarajan Yesudian and Elisabeth Haich. New York: Harper & Row, Perennial Library, 1965.

22. *Yoga Self-Taught,* by Andre van Lysebeth. New York: Barnes & Noble, 1973.

23. *Let's Do Yoga,* by Ruth Richards and Joy Abrams. New York: Holt, Rinehart and Winston, 1975. *Note:* This is a book of yoga for children, with appropriate illustrations.

24. *Be a Frog, a Bird, or a Tree: Rachel Carr's Creative Yoga Exercises for Children,* by Rachel Carr. Garden City, New York: Doubleday & Co., 1973.

25. *"Easy Does It" Yoga (for People over 60),* by Alice Christensen and David Rankin. Cleveland: Saraswati Studio, 1975.

26. *Yoga: Physical Education,* by Shri Yogendra. Bombay: The Yoga Institute, 1928. Reprinted 1974.

VII. Pranayama (Pranayama is also treated in a number of the titles listed under "Hatha Yoga")

1. *The Science of Pranayama,* by Sri Swami Sivananda. 9th ed. Sivanandanagar, India: The Divine Life Society, 1971.

2. *Pranayama,* by Swami Kuvalayananda. 5th ed. Bombay: Popular Prakashan, 1972.

3. *Science of Breath: A Complete Manual of the Oriental Breathing Philosophy,* by Yogi Ramacharaka. Chicago: Yogi Publication Society, 1905.

4. *Bragg System of Super-Brain Breathing,* by Paul C. Bragg. Burbank, California: Health Science, no date.

VIII. Alternative Approaches, Including Jogging, Dance, Sport, and Games

1. *The Complete Jogger,* by Jack Bettern. New York: Harcourt Brace Jovanovich, 1977.

2. *Beyond Jogging: The Innerspaces of Running,* by Mike Spino. Millbrae, California: Celestial Arts, 1976.

3. *The Complete Runner,* by the Editors of *Runner's World.* Mountain View, California: World Publications, 1977.

4. *Makko-Ho: Five Minutes' Physical Fitness,* by Haruka Nagai. San Francisco: Japan Publications, 1972.

5. *T'ai Chi Ch'uan: Eight Simple Chinese Exercises for Health,* by Yang Ming-shih. Tokyo: Shufunotomo, 1974.

6. *Embrace Tiger, Return to Mountain: The Essence of T'ai Chi,* by Al Chung-liang Huang. Moab, Utah: Real People Press, 1973.

7. *T'ai-Chi: The "Supreme Ultimate" Exercise for Health, Sport, and Self-Defense,* by Cheng Man-ch'ing and Robert W. Smith. Rutland, Vermont: Charles E. Tuttle, 1967.

8a. *T'ai Chi Ch'uan and I Ching,* by Da Liu. New York: Harper & Row, 1972.

8b. *Taoist Health Exercise Book,* by Da Liu. New York: Links Books, 1974.

9a. *What Is Aikido?,* by Koichi Tohei. Tokyo: Rikugei Publishing House, 1974.

9b. *Aikido in Daily Life,* by Koichi Tohei. Tokyo: Rikugei Publishing House, 1972.

9c. *Book of Ki: Co-ordinating Mind and Body,* by Koichi Tohei. Tokyo: Japan Publications, 1976.

10. *The Kung Fu Exercise Book: Health Secrets of Ancient China,* by Michael Minick. New York: Bantam Books, 1975.

11. *Introduction to Spiritual Dance and Walk.* From the work of Murshid Samuel L. Lewis. Novato, California: Prophecy Pressworks, 1972.

12a. *The Dancer Prepares: Modern Dance for Beginners,* by James Penrod and Janice Gudde Plastino. Palo Alto, California: National Press Books, 1970.

12b. *Movement for the Performing Artist,* by James Penrod. Palo Alto, California: Mayfield Publishing Company, 1974.

13. *The Ultimate Athlete,* by George Leonard. New York: Avon Books, 1977.

14. *Enjoying Gymnastics,* by the Diagram Group. New York: Paddington Press, 1976.

15. *Aquabics: Recreation and Fitness in Water,* by Richard Lough and David Stinson. New York: Harper & Row, 1973.

16. *The New Games Book.* Edited by Andrew Fluegelman. San Francisco: Headlands Press, 1976.

17. *Handbook of Recreational Games.* Compiled by Neva L. Boyd. New York: Dover Publications, 1975.

18. *The Great American Book of Sidewalk, Stoop, Dirt, Curb, and Alley Games,* by Fred Ferretti. New York: Workman Publishing Company, 1975.

19. *Everybody's a Winner: A Kid's Guide to New Sports and Fitness,* by Tom Schneider. Boston: Little, Brown and Company, 1976.

20. *The Inner Game of Tennis,* by W. Timothy Gallwey. New York: Random House, 1974.

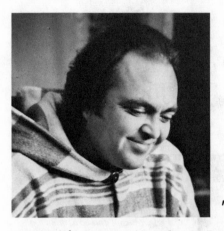

True religion,

or true life, is conscious death. It is a feeling relaxation of the whole body-mind, not just of the flesh. It is not suicide, but it is motiveless surrender in , of, and as every moment of experience. It is present release of fear, self, mind, and body, including all worlds and all relations, into the Unknown and Unknowable wherein we are appearing. It is not self-possession and psychic fasci-. nation, but it is love, peace, clarity, and embrace of Truth. When this heroic sacrifice is made with un-obstructed feeling, the Great Bliss appears, beyond birth and death, even while we are living.

Come and live this Way with me, and our God will be proved to you beyond all doubting.

—Bubba Free John

This Way of Life begins with consideration of the written Teaching of Bubba Free John.

The written Teaching
of Bubba Free John

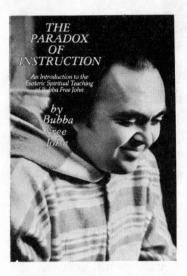

THE PARADOX OF INSTRUCTION

An Introduction to the Esoteric Spiritual Teaching of Bubba Free John 2d ed., revised and expanded

Here Bubba Free John fully presents his critical and liberating argument and describes the technical, esoteric principles of the four stages of the Way of Divine Ignorance, or Radical Understanding. He shows how this discipline of radical happiness is founded from the beginning in the intuition of Truth— and how it ultimately duplicates and transcends all the conventional or conditional realizations of yogis, saints, and sages in the great spiritual traditions.

$10.95 cloth, $5.95 paper

BREATH AND NAME

The Initiation and Foundation Practices of Free Spiritual Life

This essential companion volume to *The Paradox of Instruction* communicates the specific practices of the Way of Divine Ignorance. Bubba shows how the devotional practice of ordinary disciplines (including "conscious exercise" and other life-practices) leads naturally into simple but profound enjoyment of specific spiritual disciplines which he has called the Breath of God and the Name of God. The foundation of the whole Way is heart-felt Communion with God as all-pervading Presence, which is Gracefully and spontaneously initiated in the Company of the Spiritual Master.

$10.95 cloth, $5.95 paper

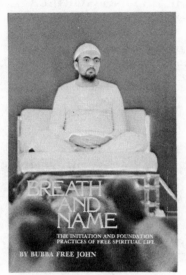

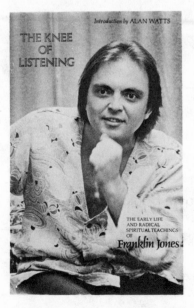

THE KNEE OF LISTENING

The Early Life and Radical Spiritual Teachings of Bubba Free John (Franklin Jones)

In his early autobiography and original essays on spiritual life in Truth, Bubba Free John shows how the whole Way that he teaches was awakened and tested beyond all doubt in his own early life. He describes the Condition of Enlightenment as he enjoyed it at birth, his years of testing and transformation as a disciple of a number of teachers, both Eastern and Western, and his ultimate restoration to the perfect illumination of Divine Ignorance, or Radical Understanding. Bubba's essays in Part II interpret this Revelation with respect to all the spiritual and worldly traditions of the great search of man.

$7.95 cloth, $3.95 paper

Forthcoming titles include:

THE EATING GORILLA COMES IN PEACE

The Principle of Love Applied to Diet and the Discipline of True Health. A Natural, Integrated Science of Whole Body Wisdom, Practiced by the World's Great Traditional Cultures and Adapted for Modern Men and Women, Especially Those Engaged in Religious or Spiritual Life.

THE ILLUSION OF OTHERS

On the Sacrifice of Subjectivity and on the Bodily Recollection of Infinity.

LOVE OF THE TWO-ARMED FORM:

The Regenerative Function of Sexuality, in Ordinary Life and in Religious or Spiritual Practice.

THE TRANSPARENT CHURCH

An Introduction to the Moral and Religious Practices of the Way of Divine Communion, the First Stage of the Way of Divine Ignorance Taught by Bubba Free John.

Preparation, revelation and the initiation of spiritual responsibility in the first stage of the Way of Divine Ignorance taught by Bubba Free John.

THE GOD OF THE WHOLE BODY

The Practical Religious and Spiritual Teaching of Bubba Free John.

A general introduction to the Teaching and work of Bubba Free John.

All books are available at fine bookstores, or from the Dawn Horse Book Depot.

Vision Mound Ceremony is continually producing other significant and basic texts by Bubba Free John. For a description of current titles, tapes and other media, please write to:

**The Dawn Horse Book Depot
P.O. Box 3680
Clearlake Highlands, Ca. 95422**

When ordering direct, please add 75c for shipping charges.
California residents please add 6% sales tax.